Praise for *Plan for Aging Well*

"Erickson's first line describes the plain reality, 'We are doing aging wrong.' And she explains why in ample, stark examples from her years of social work experience, charting the realities we all face or will face. But her real magic is her kitchen table, practical advice about how to do aging right in a world that doesn't make it easy. She provides a life-saving map to navigate the disorienting terrain virtually all of us will have to pass through."

— Charlie Sabatino, Director, ABA Commission on Law and Aging

"Erickson provides a no nonsense portrayal of the painful and neglected aspects of aging. She shares her first hand experiences in a deeply humanistic manner and challenges our acceptance of 'the normal.' She entreats us to respect the rich personal history of each individual and to work collaboratively toward a better plan for aging which incorporates physical, mental, and spiritual needs. Full of vignettes that resonate, as well as practical suggestions, Erickson shows us how we each have a role to play in improving the aging experience for ourselves and our loved ones."

— Dr. Sharon Cohen, MD, FRCPC, Director, Toronto Memory Program; Assistant Professor, University of Toronto, Division of Neurology and the Graduate Department of Speech Language Pathology; Consultant Neurologist, North York General Hospital

"This book is a helpful manual for healthcare professionals and families alike. Ms. Erickson provides a beacon of information to guide aging individuals and their families through a process that often has multiple twists and turns. This book opened my eyes as a physician to the challenges and tribulations that are often felt by patients and their caregivers, and has provided me with optimism about how I will approach elder care with my patients."

— Dr. Elise Levinoff, MD, FRCPC, Geriatric Medicine, Jewish General Hospital; Assistant Professor, Faculty of Medicine, McGill University; Internal Medicine Site Program Director, Jewish General Hospital

"Written from a social worker's perspective, *Plan for Aging Well* helps professionals, caregivers, family and friends approach supporting an older person from a place of empathy rather than a place of burden. Erickson reminds us of the potentially deeper issues that help explain why so often we as a society come up short in the care for older people when they need it. I was so glad to see the last chapter of Erickson's work where she reminds us of the specific social identities older people have, such as identifying as LGBTQ. For some reason, many care professionals and even family members discount that older people are more than their bodies. I look forward to bringing this text into social work curricula for future students to learn from, but it is truly an accessible resource for all!"

— Lauren Snedeker, DSW, LSW, LMSW, Assistant Professor of Teaching, Coordinator for the Aging and Health Certificate Program, School of Social Work, Rutgers, the State University of New Jersey

"Stephanie Erickson's book is a wake-up call for all of us. Planning for aging, including legal planning, is critical. Ms. Erickson reminds us that equally important is talking about your plans, values, beliefs and wishes with those who you designate to make decisions for you in the event that you cannot. I see the value of advance collaboration time and again in my law practice."

— Areta Lloyd, Lawyer, Estates, Trusts & Capacity Litigation

"I was engaged in this book from beginning to end. It details how our society neglects to foresee the financial, legal, emotional and spiritual aspects of aging and how we can easily plan for this season in life rather than have it fall upon us as a crisis where we no longer have any decision-making power given the emergency (i.e. loss of a spouse, a fall, loss of autonomy). I felt it was so current with what our generation and our parents are dealing with, the current state of facilities and the harsh reality of where we will end up if we do not prepare and plan for aging while we have our faculties. Such an amazing and informative read. I would **definitely** recommend this to anyone who is aging, has aging parents or works with our geriatric / assisted living/ dementia care facility."

— Sabrina Dion, R.N., Resident Care Director

"Stephanie delivers a daunting foretelling of the emotional, physical and financial toll taken in caring for elderly family members, coupled with practical applications for those embarking on this journey. Her first-hand experience gives the reader insight into the systemically poor conditions in many senior facilities. We have a responsibility to demand better, more comprehensive care in treating the whole individual with respect and dignity. Whether your elderly parent will be at home with you or in a residence, the bottom line is that it is vital to begin the conversation about aging well NOW! This book will help you develop a plan and build a solid team of support and expertise."

— Nancy, daughter and caregiver

"Stephanie has written a very poignant book giving the reader a clear picture of aging from a perspective inside an elder's mind. From that viewpoint, she offers a plethora of ideas to create a team that matches an elder's unique care needs. She has an excellent understanding of all the issues and her book is a must read!"

— Stuart Furman, Esq., Elder Law Attorney, Author of *The ElderCare Ready Book*

"Stephanie provides, with frightening accuracy, how seniors are being forgotten. 'Out of sight, out of mind' is no longer acceptable. She does, however, give us hope and steps to move in the right direction to provide our elderly with the care and respect they deserve. This book truly offers step-by-step guidelines to aging well. A how-to book for all adult children who are struggling to take care of their aging parents. These are tools that we can use ourselves to be better prepared for our, hopefully, golden years."

— Sandra, daughter and caregiver

"A very clearly written book about the challenges faced by people who are aging. This book offers insights, tangible suggestions and points that we all should consider for the future. I have worked with the aging population for many years and the experiences described by Ms. Erickson are accurate and well-described. The humour and examples used make the book a very enjoyable read and easy to understand. A must read for everyone and one that I will recommend to all of my clients."

— Mandy Novak-Leonard, MSW, social worker

"The clarity and emotion with which Stephanie writes this book provide an honest opinion and depiction of our elderly and many of their lives in assisted living residences. As an occupational therapist, I appreciated her perspective and association of an individual's past experiences with their physical, psychological, emotional and spiritual well-being. Her message that we need to do better for our elderly, and that we need to have a team of people to attend to their well-being, is not only timely but absolutely truthful."

— Susan Sofer, Occupational Therapist and Director of Autonomy Community Therapy ACT Inc.

"*Plan for Aging Well* is a great book to help you navigate the challenges that you may face caring for a loved one. As a graduate of recreational therapy and years of experience in Dementia care, I appreciate that each chapter brings a very clear understanding on how to navigate the difficult aspects of aging to ensure your loved one ages with care, dignity and pride. Stephanie brings in her own personal experience which allows you to feel connected to her as the author and relate even more to the information being shared."

— Trisha Felgar, B.A, Recreational Therapist

"Despite being something we can all expect to experience, conversations about aging, illness, and dying are often avoided by individuals and their families, leading to unfortunate and avoidable consequences for all. Advocating a 'team' approach to planning for future care, *Plan for Aging Well* will prove useful to anyone wishing to be better prepared for their later years, or better equipped to support someone they care for."

— April Hayward, MSW, Educator at Vanier College

"This book blew open my mind how as a community and system we have failed our elders. It's emotional and thought-provoking yet provides practical ways we can support our undervalued seniors who have done so much for our society. I especially love the holistic approach of practical ways we can honor and support the aging population's mind, body, and soul. This has also addressed my personal fears of aging to where I can now embrace it with more ease, grace, and preparedness. Thank you, Stephanie, for your passion, gifts, and the much-needed work you are doing for this community and world."

— Minerva Maharajh, Certified Spiritual Life Coach, Author, Teacher, and founder of Goddess of Wisdom Spiritual Life Coaching

"Stephanie Erickson takes the reader through an informative and at times personal experience on aging in today's world. As a mother, daughter and nurse, I was triggered to re-examine what I want for myself in my later years, and more so how to help my patients identify and express what really matters to them."

— Georgia Papadopoulos, RN, BScN

"It is clear that Stephanie is a fierce and passionate advocate for dignified and person-directed approaches to care. She asks the tough questions and sparks meaningful conversations that are long overdue in long-term care. I found myself cheering throughout and appreciate her ability to get to the heart of eldercare today and for the future. This book is a must for policy makers and professional and family care partners."

— Michelle Olson, PhD, LCAT, ATR-BC, ACC/MC, Gerontologist, Creative Arts Therapist, Aging and Dementia Consultant

Plan for
Aging
Well

Building a Team to Provide Physical, Emotional and Spiritual Support as We Age

Plan for Aging Well

Stephanie Erickson
MSW, LCSW

Platform Publishing, Inc.

Published by Platform Publishing, Inc.

ISBN (paperback): 978-1-7356517-0-5
ISBN (ebook): 978-1-7356517-1-2

Edited by Debra Englander and David Aretha
Publishing consultation by Martha Bullen, Bullen Publishing Services
Cover and interior design by Christy Collins, Constellation Book Services

Printed in the United States of America

This book is dedicated to my clients and their families who, throughout the years, opened their hearts and homes to me. I will be forever grateful for all you taught me about vulnerability, honesty, trust, love, sacrifice, loyalty, and resilience.

Contents

Author's Note

Throughout the book I use different terms to describe a long-term environment in which seniors live. Most often, I use the term "residence" or "nursing home."

Living environments for seniors who need light to full assistance may be referred to by different names in different countries, and those names, depending on the region, are associated with different levels of care. You may use the term "skilled nursing home," or "board and care," or "assisted living environment," or "assisted living community," or another term in your region. Please refer to the glossary at the end of this book for more information.

For all intents and purposes, I use "residence" and "nursing home" to describe residences designed for seniors who require assistance.

In addition, access to different types of services, the terms used for these services, and the fees associated will be unique to your country and region. Consult with a professional in your area to learn the specifics of how these services apply to you.

Foreword

I am an elder law attorney and after 35 years of practicing law in Southern California, I thought I knew everything about eldercare. Boy, was I wrong!

I met Stephanie online through social media. I was interested in her TEDx speech, "If we are what we say, why don't we say something different?" in which she shared her personal struggles with anxiety and how she learned, through the flying trapeze, how to tackle her negative self-talk to manage her anxiety. I really respected her aggressively attacking it by pursuing this unusual sport and I told her so.

We continued dialogues on social media where I commented on many of her posts, often starting a thread of postings, and realized that we were professionally of like mind. Occasionally a topic drew hundreds of other comments, which was gratifying since our topic was valued by so many others.

After practicing law for so many years, I considered myself an insider and thought I knew more about eldercare than most. However, when my own parents and in-laws got sick and each traveled on their eldercare journey, I realized how ignorant I really was of many practical and logistical aspects of eldercare.

I recognized that if I was that blind to the realities of eldercare, then many others were also. This revelation inspired my books *The Eldercare Ready Book* and *The ElderCare Ready Pack*.

However, after reading Stephanie's book, *Plan for Aging Well*, I grasped that I was still significantly unenlightened about the elders that I was serving.

Competent caregiving requires a comprehensive understanding of eldercare. This knowledge gives the caregiver power and solace to know that they are managing the eldercare at a high level. Knowledge and understanding equals power, competence, confidence and reduced stress and anxiety. In my experience, family members consistently have the best interests of the elder at heart. Caregivers must appreciate their role in not only managing their loved one's physical needs but also providing for their psychological and emotional support.

Caregivers must also know there is no right or wrong answer with eldercare, just an educated choice among often imperfect options. I believe that the lack of an absolute answer to the decisions to be made causes the most strife and dissention within families.

It is so clear to me that the issue of medical treatment and life sustaining care when an aging loved one is suffering is not well understood or discussed. When a crisis arises, families are often in disagreement as to what is the best choice to make. I experienced this firsthand when my parents were ill. I was of the opinion that quality of life was an important factor in determining what treatment to provide or not to provide to my parents. I looked at success rates and life expectancy after treatment, as well as the trauma of the treatment. If we went forward with a treatment, what condition were we curing them into? Another family member looked at life as always being better than death, even if the "cure" led to what I considered a horrible condition.

The last 6 months of my mother's life were the toughest that I had to live through. Life and death decisions fell upon us every day and not providing treatment meant saying goodbye. It was also very difficult to separate myself from making decisions that I wanted vs. what my mother would have wanted. The emotional element of these decisions always got in the way. In hindsight, it would have been beneficial for my entire family to have a clear understanding of my parents' expectations.

I also remember my mother often calling me at midnight and telling me I needed to come over and calm down my father who had dementia. In the background I heard him yelling at my mother saying he was leaving the assisted living home. Somehow, I managed to save myself the 45-minute drive to see him in person by talking with him on the phone. I am not a psychologist and had difficulty with how to deal with his outbursts. I think I just got lucky. It also didn't help that he was a psychiatrist, so I knew that, even with his dementia, he was out of my league.

In my many years of practice, I have seen families struggle with complex care issues, facility choices, medicine management, the elder's safety, physician visits and meetings, the elder's finances and taxes, family meetings, continuous monitoring of independent caregivers, quality of care issues in facilities, and much more. It was, and is, quite overwhelming.

Stephanie hits a home run by having her readers put themselves into the shoes of elders so as to understand their whole self. Her descriptions of the care industry are shocking, depressing, and show how disgraceful living conditions can be in those "golden years." In her book, she shows readers very effectively what it's like to be an elder and how elders are affected by the care provided. She offers valuable tools and advice to address this paradigm. And, writing from her own experiences, Stephanie relates an abundance of stories from her practice to bring her points home.

Although the Canadian and U.S. medical systems differ, there are two universal truths: 1. People get old, ill and die; 2. The medical community cannot change rule number 1. All they can do is extend the journey and hopefully make it more enjoyable. However, our medical systems must better address quality of life, not simply emphasize the financial costs of extending life. More books need to be written to address these issues and provide a foundation for sparking change in the care of our elders. Until then we must learn from as many experts and sources available.

Stephanie is a talented and experienced social worker, family caregiving expert, media commentator and columnist. She was guest commentator for years on "Breakfast Television" based in Montreal on Rogers TV, hosted "Caregiver's Circle," a web talk radio series on which I was her guest, and was co-host of "Life Unrehearsed" on CJAD800, Montreal's largest talk radio station. In addition, she has hosted multiple web series related to caregiving. She is also a keynote speaker and provides trainings to the financial, legal and financial industries, as well as to community groups on how to assist older adults. She currently runs a clinical practice in which she conducts decision-making capacity evaluations in legal proceedings for individuals with dementia. This background and her vast professional experience form the bedrock of her book. And, like me, she found a calling to write a book to help others with their eldercare journeys.

Stephanie's expertise and experience with elders' emotional and psychological needs and the information and insights she shares in this book have given me a real education and will assist me tremendously in my elder law practice. I was honored to preview an early draft of her book and truly blessed to have been asked to write this Foreword.

I hope you find this book as interesting, enlightening, and educational as I did. Caregivers need to have their eyes opened as to what caregiving means and how to effectively give care to a loved one. They are vulnerable souls and you are their protector, provider, confidant, and caregiver to make their Golden Years as golden as they can be.

I hope you appreciate Stephanie's book as much as I did. It is a valuable resource which I will give to all of my clients.

Stuart Furman, Esq.
Author of *The ElderCare Ready Book* and *The ElderCare Ready Pack*
ElderCare Ready, LLC
Southern California Legal Center, Inc.

Introduction

We are doing aging wrong. I see it every day in my work as a social worker. Families aren't proactively having discussions about their expectations of care and treatment. Legal documents aren't prepared. Residences are understaffed and based on a medical model that completely ignores our whole being. Seniors at home are isolated and at ongoing risk of falls, malnutrition, medication mishaps, abuse, and neglect.

Almost every time I enter a nursing home I am hit with the stench of pain, suffering, and urine. I see human beings lined up in their wheelchairs while a television broadcasting *The View* plays loudly in the background. Most residents are hunched over asleep, completely disengaged from anything happening around them. Staff cannot be found.

When I ask staff about my patient—*How is she doing? What are her medical problems? How involved is the family?*—too often the staff has no answers. Sometimes they don't even know who the patient is. I don't blame them. They have so many sick people to care for and are working on auto-pilot just trying to get enough people washed, cleaned, and to the breakfast table on time. Families are left out of treatment decisions and are wracked with guilt over the reality that their own personal and work demands leave them unable to do more.

I am scared out of my mind to get old.

Exposed

The seeds of this book were planted in 2013. I took a stab at writing a book on aging, but raising young kids and a busy clinical practice took over and the book became an unopened folder on my desktop. In October 2019 I decided that I could no longer wait to speak out and fight for change and I began to write again. By mid-February 2020, the book was mostly done.

Enter the pandemic.

It pains me to say that I'm not surprised that COVID-19 has taken so many lives of seniors. This population is highly vulnerable, and illness is one of the things that can impact a senior dramatically. When a run-of-the-mill gastrointestinal infection or flu enters a residence, it rapidly spreads and we lose lives to even mild strains of viruses.

Why is that? Seniors' immune systems are not as robust as they once were and they are further compromised by underlying health problems. Residences do not provide staff with ample, appropriate protective equipment. Staff are not always trained in infection control procedures, or due to time restraints (as a result of poor staff ratios), they do not have the time to take all the necessary steps and are forced to cut corners. Staff are undervalued and poorly paid, so many are compelled to take shifts at multiple nursing homes, transferring illness from one location to another.

> **As COVID-19 entered the scene the entire world was awakened to the significant flaws in our healthcare system, housing systems, and community support for seniors.**

Knowing what we do about seniors and their needs, it astounds me that there were not proactive steps taken to mitigate the devastation that COVID-19 presented. In theory, if government and nursing home owners actually acknowledged the shortcomings in our care structure and delivery, they would have been over-prepared for something like COVID-19. These homes would have had arsenals of personal protective equipment on hand and staff would not have fallen ill and had to stay home—or worse, lose their own lives.

If staff ratios had been acceptable prior to the pandemic, seniors would have received immediate care and attention instead of being left, in some cases, for days without anyone tending to their needs. If staff were valued and well paid for the incredible service they provide to this population, they wouldn't have been working in multiple locations and spreading the virus.

Family caregivers wouldn't have been completely isolated from their loved ones trapped in these death chambers, which many of the nursing homes became. The seniors who were already isolated, alone, and afraid wouldn't have suffered further loneliness and fear as they were suddenly cut off from their family and friends. Staff didn't have an extra moment to phone families to relay an update on their loved one's health, and this created a panic for families.

I have known for years that our system is failing our seniors. We treat those who gave our country everything as if their lives don't matter now that they can no longer "contribute." Seniors are seen as "bodies" and measured in "tasks" and "care hours" instead of as living, breathing souls. Staff to patient ratios are unacceptably low. Care is focused on the body, and the mind and soul are neglected. Some private pay homes are, at the end of a day, a business, a corporation. At times, the human component is lost. More attention is given to appearances—the bells and whistles like beautiful lobbies—to attract new customers. So, instead of allocating resources for care or better staff salaries and conditions, the revenue is directed with a marketing angle or to fill the pockets of the shareholders. Funding is sparse in the public sectors and dollars don't make their way down to front-line staff and resident resources.

We live in a medical model of reactivity in which very little is planned out, step by step, taking the whole person into consideration. This model does not look at each person as a holistic being with emotional, psychological, and spiritual needs as well as physical needs. It rarely considers how powerful the mind/body connection is. It neglects the opportunity to value our whole self—mind, body, and soul—and by doing so it contributes to the decline of our overall physical health.

Instead, our current healthcare system is disease focused. It identifies a problem and endeavors to fix it. If you have physical pain, the medical model jumps in to make a diagnosis, prescribe a medication or intervention, or perform a surgery. This model forgets to evaluate the other parts of who we are. It doesn't consider that perhaps another area needs attention, and if those were attended to, our physical health might improve.

Now Is the Time

When it comes to aging, most of us would rather run the other way. We're afraid to get old and die. So, what do most sane people do when they're afraid of something? They avoid it. I get that. I do it too. But our ignorance is not sparking bliss. It's leading to hopelessness, depression, financial hardships, isolation, and stress.

If you were going to design a kitchen, wouldn't you spend endless hours searching online for images to reproduce in your home? Perhaps you would hire a professional for advice. You would take time to go through paint colors, tile, and floor samples; shop for the right appliances; buy a new dishware; and purchase a table and chairs to match. You would carefully think out how every inch of your space can accommodate, with precision, your cookie sheets in an orderly, upright fashion—your drawers sliding out slowly, your cabinets with shelves on rollers for easy access, etc. You would make sure that every nook and cranny of the kitchen design fits your specific needs. We need to approach aging as we approach designing a kitchen.

> *Plan for Aging Well* is focused on this concept:
> We must consider the big picture of what we want to
> achieve as we grow older while paying special attention
> to each nook and cranny of our being—our physical,
> spiritual, social, emotional, psychological, and financial
> self—in order to design a plan that fits with our own
> personal values, expectations, and hopes.

I wrote this book because we must prepare and be proactive about our future, and I want to do my part to contribute to the solution. As a society, we cannot afford to wait another minute to change the way we support an increasingly aging population. We've all heard that the aging tsunami is coming. We have no time to waste.

The population is aging and soon our seniors will outnumber those who can take care of them. According to the U.S. Census Bureau projections, by 2030 one in five Americans will be a senior citizen, and by 2050 they will account for approximately 25 percent of the population. In Canada, by 2030 seniors will make up 23 percent of the nation. We all know that the future of an overburdened healthcare system, a lack of sustainable resources, and an exhausted family system will break, and it is the families who will be there to try to catch the breaking pieces and find glue strong enough to hold them together.

If I'm honest, part of my motivation is selfish. I don't want to be left to rot and die in this system that our governments and society have built. I am no fool. I know the later years of life are not "golden." At fifty years old, I feel the aches and pains, see my mobility and energy changing, and know that in many ways, life gets harder.

But, I also know better now. My experience as a social worker (and human) has shown me that despite our physical changes, we are still alive. The human, spiritual, and emotional parts of us don't lose their luster. In fact, the depth of our soul and mind become even more valuable and in need of love and attention. As our bodies need more time to sit still, our minds and souls need more stimulation and time to reflect and process what is behind us and what is yet to come.

Ageism is real. Our society devalues humans when they are perceived as no longer productive and vital. We are all about "doing" and being "busy" and "accomplishments," and as our bodies age, we are slower to do and accomplish in the most traditional of definitions, so the world leaves us behind. We push older adults aside as if it weren't their aching backs that built the modern world in which we flourish.

> **All individuals of any age are an integral part of society and deserve to be valued and respected.**

The Pathway to Change

With every challenge, every heartache, every tragedy there is an opportunity. I am sickened at what has happened to our seniors with this pandemic, as I'm sure you are. So, what can we do about it?

The tendency will be for residence owners and governmental bodies to increase the patient-staff ratios and pat themselves on the back for doing something. I'm not arguing that this is not a great step but it will not solve the deeper issue. Our seniors need more than a person to push their wheelchair from point A to point B.

Seniors need a community of healthcare professionals and family caregivers to care for their whole being. Professionals must have training that includes attention to the body, mind, and soul. This training must come not only from the organizations that employ these staff, but from the educational institutions that structure the curriculum that develops a professional's basic approach to care. The team of professionals and family must be well-informed of the patient's right to choose their goals and objectives and work in collaboration to meet these goals and to hold each other accountable if focus is lost.

> **We don't need to put band-aids over an already broken system. We need real change and that only comes with a complete rebuild.**

My hope is that this book wakes up a sleeping society and its "business as usual" system. I want society to change the way it approaches aging and learn how to respect and celebrate the wholeness of who we are as human beings so that the type of care and support we offer matches that wholeness. Family caregivers and seniors can use this book as a guide to apply pressure to our healthcare system, demanding the system step up and make things right.

This book is also meant to inspire healthcare professionals

who support seniors to dig deep and ask themselves hard questions. Do I see the person in front of me as a unique and whole person? Am I working in collaboration with other professionals? Is my patient's voice heard? Is the family a part of my care plan? Can I do more?

Although this book was based on my pre-pandemic experiences, the ideas pave the pathway for real change in a current and post-pandemic world. Let's use our current global health crisis as an opportunity to demolish and fully reconstruct our system and how we approach aging and care.

Don't get me wrong. I have seen amazing care delivered by top-notch professionals. I have seen staff with the patience of angels soflty encourage a scared senior to stand up out of a wheelchair. I have known nurses to share details about a patient's life that tell me how much time has been spent really learning about the person. Many times I have seen an approach to care adjusted, and adjusted again as the staff discover new and better ways to meet the needs of a person. Unfortunately, those times surprise me more than what I describe in this book.

This book describes what I've seen as the normal (sub) standard care. I share stories of my observations and experiences to demonstrate the depth of our failures. Why do I do this? For a few reasons. One, I want you to feel the pain and heartache. If it hits you deep and hard and makes you angry and sad, I've done my job. Most long-lasting changes only come after we've hit rock bottom and, in my mind, we have. Second, learning of our current failures is an essential step to ensure that we have a clear lens on what exactly is missing so we avoid repeating our mistakes. We must fully understand our history in order to move beyond it and create a new and vibrant approach to caring for seniors.

Each chapter addresses a different aspect of aging—the mind, the body, the heart and soul, and the pocketbook. I share examples of what each of these areas looks like in someone's life and within our current healthcare and family systems. I also offer some quick and easy examples of how, with minimal effort, we can completely flip the way we care for someone. Finally, the concept of team caregiving is explained. Each team member is presented and their role defined. Examples of how beneficial a collaborative approach can be are explored.

I can only hope that something good comes out of this pandemic nightmare and, at some point, we return to normalcy. But in terms of senior care, I don't want us to return to what was once considered normal. It was and is unacceptable.

Let's do better.

CHAPTER 1

The Problem

"My mom is getting older."

"My dad is losing his memory."

"My grandmother is no longer able to drive safely."

All of these statements are about one person—a mother, a father, a grandmother. This is how our society describes those who are aging and this is the driving force behind how our healthcare and support systems generally intervene. The semantics and practical responses to aging endorse a perception that we age in isolation.

A woman named Susan visits her family physician, Dr. Cook, with her daughter, Annie, who waits anxiously in the waiting room. After the exam with Susan, Dr. Cook calls his patient's daughter into his office and asks to meet with her alone. Dr. Cook looks at Annie and says, "Your mother needs support at home. You need to arrange something," and then Susan and her daughter are sent on their way.

I understand. The doctor is treating his patient, not the family. But does this type of advice really work? Now Susan is left wondering what was said to her daughter and she is feeling vulnerable, scared, and isolated. Annie is feeling overwhelmed and alone and she is at a loss as to where to start "arranging something" for her mother. Who is going to pay for this assistance and what actual assistance does she need? This scenario doesn't provide a solution that would allow a senior to be open to accepting help from others or for an adult child to feel competent to take on the role of a caregiver. Susan is not aging in isolation with her daughter as a peripheral member of her life. They are aging together, and the doctor providing care should recognize this reality and provide relevant advice and help. The doctor could have discussed ideas such as home care services or day programs that could support Susan's mom. The doctor could have given Susan a referral to a caregiver's support group so she could find some support and resources from others in her same situation. One would assume that physicians have a database filled with resources at the tips of their fingers and instinctually link patients and their families with appropriate support. Often, it's just not the case.

> **We age as a team, and it takes a team to cope and to manage the challenges (and joys) of aging. Our team consists of all of us—our parents, our children, other relatives, neighbors, the members of our healthcare system, and our work environments.**

Due to the inherent strain caused by a lack of resources, shortage of funds, and in some regions a lack of qualified staff, our health, medical, and community care services cannot meet the demands of the aging population. Therefore, the burden of care falls on the family.

Even our semantics of aging are isolating. Take, for example, the word "burden," which I intentionally used. It's a term used to describe the result of caring for another person, and one that, in its meaning alone, creates a perception of negativity. What does this say about how we approach aging?

We must remember that most family caregivers do not have the luxury (if you call the responsibilities of caregiving a luxury) to manage this responsibility full time. In fact, according to AARP, 61 percent of caregivers were employed at some point in the last year while they were simultaneously caregiving (Caregiving in the U.S. 2020 Report, AARP). Caregivers are working and organizing medical appointments, making meals, cleaning the home, managing medication, reviewing financial statements, and assisting their parents with personal hygiene care. All of these tasks are somehow accomplished over the weekend, after work, or during work hours (to the disapproval of the employer—another member of the team). Often these family caregivers have their own children—other team members—for whom they need to be available.

Yet, few people want to talk about the responsibilities of helping our families and the control of our aging process. We complain about the system and the lack of funding or efficient policies. We complain to our friends about our children neglecting us or about our parents who refuse to accept help. Instead of everyone voicing similar grievances, imagine if we all understood the continuum of aging and how each experience, transition, and crisis comes with a ricochet impact on all team members. Wouldn't this perspective promote team aging?

If my mother falls ill and I have to fly to California to assist her for a month, will my employer give me time off? Will it be unpaid? If it is unpaid, how will I pay my monthly bills? Will I have my job when I return? Do I have to take money from my retirement account to cover the flight and a hotel since I can't stay at my mother's retirement home? How will my husband manage his job (which involves travel) and our children's schedules while I am away? If he has to hire a babysitter, how will we pay for that since I will be losing my salary while I'm away?

Will my daughter have to miss her cheerleading competition? Will she be allowed to stay on the team if she misses the competition? Will my son still be able to get to his football practices after school? Will my son's grades drop and his stress level at school increase, leading to behavioral problems and an intervention by his teacher? How will my husband find the time to take his mother to do her grocery shopping if I am not available to stay with our kids? How will my mother-in-law's health suffer if my husband is not as available?

If I need medical attention when I'm in California, how will I pay for it? How can I pay for my mother's treatment since her husband is ill and is not able to manage the finances? Is there any plan in place for some type of auto-payment from her bank to the care provider on her behalf?

Phew! Do you feel overwhelmed? I do, and I haven't even asked the questions related to my mother's health, my relationship with my sister and my mother's husband, their health, their finances, etc. Look at how one aging relative's illness leads to a ricochet effect on the entire extended family. It is overwhelming; you can't say that your parents are getting older and leave it at that.

Our team lacks insight. We have doctors making decisions independently of the impact on the family. We have hospitals that treat the presenting illness but rarely address the factors that contributed to the condition or what needs to be done with regard to the ongoing management of the illness. We have a reactive medical system, not a proactive one that looks at prevention of illness and the introduction (and financial support) of preventive health and wellness programs. We have individual family members who have limited and private conversations with one another but who are not creating a family care plan. (Care plans are discussed in Chapter Seven, Team Caregiver.) We have seniors who plan financially for aging but then don't share their decisions, values, and ideas about how to use their money with any of their family members.

We are each making independent decisions instead of thinking of the role each person plays and how we can work together effectively. If our team members deconstructed aging with a clear lens, they would acknowledge the painfully obvious fact that acting as if we age alone is not working. Our medical systems are overburdened. Our financial support systems are fraying at the seams. Our families are overworked, overstressed, and exhausted.

> **We are spinning our wheels trying to evaluate and respond to one system instead of trying to transform how aging is viewed around the world.**

Statistically, most families are thrown into the ocean in a crisis with a limited plan or no plan whatsoever. The adult child is at the helm trying to navigate this huge aging ship with limited support from his or her parent's "crew."

We need to shout louder. The rooftops are not high enough. Each family, each healthcare provider, each service provider, each healthcare system, and each employer must revisit how we think about and approach aging.

CHAPTER 2

The Answer

This book challenges adult children, seniors, healthcare professionals, governmental bodies, and other private service industries to change how they think about and respond to aging. Through my experiences as a social worker, I have had a front seat view and understand the holistic approach necessary to design your aging plan. I will examine the primary situations—financial, emotional, legal, physical, logistical, cognitive, and spiritual—impacted by aging. With these personal accounts, connections are made between team members that may be otherwise ignored. Take, for example, the questions I raised earlier about what I would need to do if my mother fell ill and needed my help for one month. Many of you probably wouldn't have anticipated the ricochet impact on my family's health and financial situation.

When asked about how her family was impacted, a daughter recounted:

When my mother had her stroke the hospital team told me she was no longer able to walk safely or to perform everyday tasks such as cleaning and cooking, and she was cognitively impaired. They discharged her into my care with a list of residences.

I had to research residences and then purchase a walker and then rent a wheelchair. I arranged for a medication dispensing system that I thought would meet my mother's needs and keep her safe.

After moving her to a semi-autonomous residence—which was supposed to provide an adequate level of care and assistance—I realized within the first two weeks that she was not semi-autonomous at all. She was dependent. This was not predicted by the hospital team and there was no follow-up to help me manage this sudden discovery.

I started visiting her twice a day to make sure that she maintained her physical health by administering her medication and making her meals since I could not afford to pay the residence more money to provide more hours of care. I researched and bought a special sensor that turned off the stovetop in case she forgot.

Obviously, my work life was directly impacted. Even when I was at work I wasn't really there mentally. Unfortunately, she continued to fall. She broke her hip once, and two weeks after her return to the residence she broke her arm!

My health was not great anyway, and after I started helping my mother daily, my blood pressure increased so I had to increase my medication dosage. I told my doctor what was causing my stress but he just gave me more medication and offered no resources for the source of the problem except to tell me I should stop helping my mom so much. Then who would help her if I didn't? Certainly not my brother, who lives on the other side of the country! Plus, my stress level was so high that I was not as available for my own kids. I didn't know what to do.

My mom had signed a Living Will putting me in charge so I knew in theory she trusted me to make decisions for her. But we never talked about it. I didn't feel confident that I really knew where she wanted to live if she needed care. Did she expect me to take her to my house and hire somebody? Did she want me to hire someone to help her at the residence and for me to keep my job? Was I supposed to use her savings for the home, for private care, or for her beneficiaries? I didn't know her priorities, which I desperately wanted to respect. I was overwhelmed and confused.

This example demonstrates the missed opportunities that could have led to better responses from the team. For example, years ago the mother could have made arrangements with her financial planner to set aside an account that her daughter could access in order to pay for support and care. Although the mother put her legal papers in order, she and her daughter should have discussed in more detail how the mother wanted her money spent as well as her care priorities. This could have relieved pressure on her daughter.

The hospital team could have met with the daughter to evaluate residences instead of simply handing her a general list, which left the daughter feeling ill equipped. Or, the hospital team could have referred her to a relocation specialist who could help her evaluate several residences that would most closely meet her needs. There could have been a liaison from the hospital team to follow up with the daughter to ensure that the care in the residence was adequate and to assist the daughter in finding and purchasing the safety and ambulation items. The mother's doctor could have referred the daughter to support groups or organizations to help navigate the maze of caregiving.

This family was not aging as a team. There were team members involved—the care recipient (mother), the primary caregiver (daughter), the hospital, the residence, an attorney who created a Health Care Advanced Directive,[1] the physician—but the response of these members was to segregate the issues, rather than connect them. Each team member had their own agenda and this was the driver behind their recommendation, without considering what the senior and his or her family actually wanted or needed. *Plan for Aging Well* is aimed at inspiring individuals and healthcare, legal, and financial systems to rethink the way in which we approach aging, working to collaborate with the collective goal that the patient set, and not based on our own agendas.

I am on a mission to encourage families to start the conversation about aging now—not when there is a crisis. I hope

---

1 A Health Care Advanced Directive is one term used to describe a document in which your wishes for care and support are documented. You choose a person to represent you should you be unable to make your own decisions. These documents have different names and nuances depending on the region in which you live. This is discussed further in The Aging Pocketbook chapter.

to create a new outlook on aging as an extended family team. It is my hope that after families adopt a new perspective, they will, in turn, advocate to the professionals who serve them to rethink how aging is viewed and approached. I hope that over time these family conversations will bleed into the health, medical, legal, and financial systems so that everyone begins to view and approach aging as a team.

CHAPTER 3

The Aging Mind

I recently went to meet with a client who has dementia. This was my first time meeting this woman, and her brother and sister-in-law planned to meet me at the nursing home. My client has a son who lives in another province, and he couldn't join us. I had been to this residence before, but that didn't neutralize the shock of what I faced when I walked into the large nursing home.

As I entered the lobby, I immediately felt as though I was in a hospital when I encountered a huge, round desk in the center of the lobby. There was a man sitting behind it, looking at a screen. Perhaps he was keeping an eye on the facility, but my guess was that he was reading his email. His eyes never looked up as I approached the desk to sign in. He didn't say hello, ask me if I needed assistance, or request my identification. I could have been anyone doing anything. There seemed to be no security whatsoever.

To my left was a café, which consisted of ten tables and some chairs but no place to purchase a coffee or snack. Three tables were occupied. At two of these tables, one person in a wheelchair was asleep and another person who looked to be a companion stared at her phone as her client slept. At the third table, a man in a wheelchair interacted with a family member sitting next to him. As I walked by the café, a second man in a wheelchair was deposited and left at a table by a staff member who just walked away, not saying a word.

I rode the elevator to the second floor to meet my client and her family. Before I even arrived, the smell of urine began to permeate the elevator. When the doors slid open, the smell was so strong I had to tell my stomach contents to stay put. A sign posted outside the elevator doors showed me which direction to go. This residence was so big that it would have been easy to get lost. On each floor there must have been about fifty rooms, many with two beds to a room. I turned left and walked down a long, stark, white hallway, which lacked any color or artwork.

In front of me I could see the central area for the residents who lived on this side of the floor. As I walked closer, the sounds of the residents got louder. When I arrived at this area, I saw ten residents, all in wheelchairs dumped in front of a television with not a staff member in sight. One woman repetitively made the same sound: "Ah, oh. Ah, oh. Ah, oh." I wondered how long she had been doing this and what she was trying to say. I got my indirect answer when I saw two separate staff members walk by her without a glance. Clearly, this was a repetitive pattern that the staff were used to ignoring.

Walking further down the hallway, I passed a man with his hand straight out in front of him, as if holding a plate. He kept saying, "Help, help, help." Staff members walked by him without a word as well.

As I turned the corner, I passed an aide mopping the floor. She advised me to be careful as she had just thrown bleach on the floor and wasn't sure what liquid she was mopping up. As I passed her, I caught sight of a man roaming the hallways. The crotch and one side of his pants were soaking wet, so it was clear where the liquid on the floor had come from.

I also passed a man flopped over with his head on a table, sitting on what looked like a desk from an elementary school. When I was done with my client interview an hour later, he was still there, head on the table. I don't know if staff interacted with him during that time, but he definitely hadn't moved.

When I entered my client's room, I found her sitting alone in her wheelchair, staring at nothing, doing nothing. I wondered when the last time was that a staff member had been in to check on her. Did they notice she was staring at a blank wall?

I looked for the nurse to obtain more information about my client. Her office was so nondescript it was difficult to spot. That made me wonder how patients and families could locate the staff when they needed something. The one bright part of this day? The nurse had been working at this residence for seven years and on this particular floor for a year (this was refreshing, since turnover is so common) and she really knew my client well.

I know my description of my work sounds horrible. You're probably wondering if there are ever good experiences for someone with dementia living in a nursing home. Thankfully, there are. In some residences I'm greeted by a dog or cat. I've seen firsthand the dramatic impact animals can have on people with dementia (and so many other illnesses). I've smelled freshly made popcorn or chocolate cookies baking in the afternoon. I've seen staff singing to their clients as they administer a shower. I listen as staff call individuals by their first name, or Daddy, or doctor (whatever seems to make the person comfortable) and truly engage with individuals. I've heard music from the 1920s and '30s fill the air with joyful sound while watching a staff member dance with a patient. But unfortunately, these experiences are not the norm. Most of the time I'm disappointed, sad, disheartened, and angry with what I see.

I'm not pleased that the introduction to this chapter is so depressing, but I'm not here to sugarcoat the unpleasant truths of what I often see at nursing homes or deny the fact that dementia is in the cards for so many elderly people. Most of us will have mild cognitive impairment when we age, which does not always progress to dementia, so don't panic. But it is a reality that dementia will likely touch someone we love at some point during our time on earth.

Before we move on to the individual symptoms of dementia, we must first understand the basics.

What Is Dementia?

Dementia is the global term for a cluster of symptoms that impact various cognitive and functional abilities due to changes in our brain. There are many diseases that cause dementia.

Recently, the diagnostic manual (DSM-5, American Psychiatric Association) used by physicians and others to diagnosis neurological disorders, personality disorders, mood disorders, and more was updated. Dementia is now called a neurocognitive disorder. For simplicity and ease, I will use the term "dementia" as more people are familiar with this term. Alzheimer's is the most common type of dementia. Other types of dementia include Lewy-Body Dementia, Vascular Dementia, Korsakoff's Dementia, Frontotemporal Dementia, and many more.

There are six major categories of symptoms that are affected:

- Complex attention
- Executive functioning (planning, decision-making, judgment)
- Learning and memory
- Language
- Perceptual-motor (recognizing faces, drawing, small motor skills)
- Social cognition (recognizing emotions)

Dementia is progressive, and at present there is no cure for it. While its onset is typically slow, it progresses at varying rates depending on which type of dementia the person has. For some, dementia is caused by a vascular event, so its onset is immediate. There are only a few medications available to treat dementia. Their purpose is to slow down the progression of symptoms but they only do that for a short period of time. There are things we can all do to keep our brain sharp and our body healthy to delay or optimally avoid getting dementia. Physical exercise, nutrition, social stimulation, and cognitive stimulation are important steps to take in keeping not only our body but our mind healthy. Unfortunately, there are some genetic risks that are unavoidable.

Thinking about the possibility of suffering from dementia is unpleasant but essential in order to design a plan that fits our family values. The reality is that many of the nursing homes available are just as I described throughout this book, and caring for someone with many of the symptoms that present with this disease at home is very, very difficult. Having open discussions about the journey of dementia is essential for your family.

"It's not just my mind I'm losing"

My main clinical work is to evaluate individuals for decision-making capacity. Most of my clients have dementia. A few months ago, I interviewed a man who had moved into a long-term care residence when he could no longer care for himself. During our interview, he cried and told me he thought about suicide and expressed how depressed he felt being away from his wife.

At one point he told me he was having chest pain, so I immediately went to the nursing station. I didn't see a nurse, but there were two nurse's aides sitting in a side room. I told them about my client's chest pains. One of the aides looked at me, then at her colleague, and let out an exasperated breath. She slowly grabbed his medical chart and they begin to flip through it. When she discovered there was no medication listed for chest pains, she shrugged her shoulders and said, "Well, there's no medication."

I could not believe I had to do this, but I said to her, "Well, can someone go and see if he's okay?" She let out another sigh, slowly stood up, grabbed a blood pressure cuff, and moseyed over to his room. After taking his pressure, she turned to me and said, "It's normal."

I was incredulous at her response. I responded, "Can you alert the nurse? He was also expressing suicidal ideation and the nurse, doctor, and social worker need to know." Another sigh. She picked up her phone out of her pocket and called the nurse, then told me there was no answer but she would ask the nurse to follow up. I had my doubts this would happen. I was with the client for another thirty-five minutes and no one came to check on him.

On my way out I passed by the two nurse's aides. Guess what they were doing? They were sitting in the side room looking through a magazine. Guess what the other residents were doing? Sitting, or should I say slumping, in chairs and wheelchairs not watching the television as it blared in front of them, completely disengaged. I was furious!

My client was experiencing a pain trifecta—physical, spiritual, and emotional—and no one at the residence seemed to care. This, ladies and gentlemen, is the state of far too many long-term care residences.

Healthcare professionals often brush off people with dementia since they are confused and may not be expressing themselves clearly. It's easier (in the short term) to assume that there is no hidden meaning to be discovered behind a behavior and move on to the next task. It takes time to understand what behavior and verbal patterns may mean. Most healthcare professionals don't have the time and some don't have the desire.

It is true that people with dementia may say their knee hurts, and when the nurse comes to evaluate the pain, the person forgets they even had it. I understand that this may make it less likely for staff to believe or intervene when patients make statements. Dementia patients can be exhausting, and I know it is not easy for healthcare professionals or families to manage these symptoms. However, I believe that if our nursing homes had better staff-patient ratios, the staff would be able to spend more individualized time getting to know their patients. This would allow the care to be specific and appropriate to each person.

> **We must remember that individuals with dementia have difficulty evaluating, expressing, and ensuring their needs are met. It is up to the healthcare professionals and families to proactively assess, understand, and respond to their needs.**

There are ways for healthcare professionals to evaluate how someone with dementia is doing that have nothing to do with verbal communication. They can look at facial expressions such as grimacing or clenching one's jaw as possible pain indicators. When a person with dementia cries out when being moved into a different position, he may have pain or may be fearful or confused as to what is happening. We can get to know a person's patterns, and when there is a slight change we must take the time to investigate further to evaluate if there is an infection, or pain, or emotional, or spiritual distress so that we can properly attend to it.

"I want to go home"

Imagine waking up one morning and finding yourself in an unfamiliar bed. You get up looking for the bathroom and cannot find it. You walk aimlessly around the home not recognizing one item, yet the person walking with you keeps saying to you, "You are home. You are home." How frightening that must feel.

Disorientation to place is a very common symptom that I see often in my clinical practice. In the beginning stages of dementia many of my clients understand they are in their home, although they may not be able to tell me their address. As the disease progresses, they may deny that they are in their home and express worry and fear as to where they are. Other times, although they are sitting in Montreal in the home in which they've lived for years, they tell me they are home in Switzerland and their parents' room is upstairs.

I cannot count the number of times I have heard a story of a parent driving to a child's home, a drive a person had taken for years, and becoming completely disoriented and turned around. They drive north instead of south, crossing a bridge instead of continuing straight, or running out of gas at some point, and often the police or a good Samaritan has stepped in to help.

This disorientation to place can lead to some scary outcomes, such as people leaving their home to "go home" and then getting lost somewhere. Fortunately, there are some innovative new devices, such as a GPS insole in a shoe, that can help keep track of an individual's whereabouts. Family members or caregivers can also make adaptations to the patient's home, such as adding a lock at the top of the door that requires a key, so the person cannot wander out while a caregiver is in the shower. (There are some risks in this approach that should be discussed with a professional before you implement them.)

> **What is most important is to try to understand the feeling or place that the person is trying to convey when he or she says, "I want to go home."**

Could the person be referring to a childhood home? Or a place, in a general sense, that feels good?

Distraction is a great intervention for many symptoms of dementia. When someone you care for is disoriented and he says he "wants to go home," you can ask him to describe the home, the smell, the colors he sees, and who lives there. After asking these questions and listening to his answers, you could suggest he has a snack before leaving for the trip home. Likely, while he's eating a snack, he will forget he made this request. At a minimum, you will understand the feeling he is trying to capture in that "home" and you can try to reproduce it.

"Where is my daughter?"

Imagine you are in the shower and someone is helping you wash your body. You are completely naked and vulnerable and have no idea who this person is. If this happened to me today I would freak out. This is what happens to many individuals with a dementia diagnosis, and when they resist, they are labeled as aggressive and often given medication. Wouldn't you become aggressive if someone you didn't know was trying to take your clothes off and get you in the shower?

> **Not knowing the people who are providing care and support can be very scary for someone with dementia and can lead to outbursts and aggression.**

When someone is said to be aggressive, I twist that around in my mind and think that the person is protective, meaning that she is worried or afraid about her personal safety and is doing what she can to keep herself safe. I think if we all flip our ideas about this symptom it could help us approach and support a person differently.

This is the one symptom that I find particularly distressing. I cannot imagine my mom looking at me and not knowing who I am, or the pain that my children will feel if I do not recognize them one day. When I ask my clients if they have children and they say "no" as they are sitting next to their son or daughter, my heart breaks. No matter how much a family member can intellectualize that it's the disease doing this and a brain gone haywire, it hurts. I have never seen a caregiver ever adjust to this situation.

However, I have seen caregivers get to a place where they can manage this symptom quite well. I suggest that instead of testing a parent by asking, "Who am I?" a family member walks in the room and says, "Hi, Mom. It's Tricia, your daughter." Or when a parent is struggling to remember if she has kids and their names, a family member jumps in to give the details and generates an immediate conversation about a shared memory. I've noticed that this approach really eases the mind of my clients, takes the edge off of their feeling there was something they should have known but didn't, and reduces agitation. These seemingly small actions can lead to a far more positive interaction for both the parent and family.

Offering statements rather than questions also relieves the fear of the person with dementia that he or she is doing something wrong or is stupid for not knowing the answer. Unfortunately, in my line of work, I evaluate decision-making capacity, so it requires me to ask a lot of questions, and that may make the client feel they are put on the spot. Sometimes if I ask a client what the date is, or when his birthday is, or if she has children, I hear my client say they are "dumb" or "stupid" because they recognize they were unable to answer a very simple question.

If you are a professional, I understand that you need to ask open-ended questions. But if you are a family member, it is not your job to test somebody. It is perfectly acceptable and encouraged to give all of the details you can. For example, instead of saying, "Mom, do you remember your granddaughter? What's her name?" You can say, "Mom, your granddaughter Isabelle is here to visit you. She's ten now and is in the fourth grade and she wants to tell you about her new puppy."

"But it's morning!"

A telltale symptom of dementia is disorientation to time. This refers to a person not realizing that it's actually 2020, not 1973, or that today is Monday, not Wednesday. As with most symptoms of dementia, disorientation to time usually starts slowly. A person may think he is in 1989 instead of 2020 on one day, and then three weeks pass with not one moment of disorientation. As the disease progresses, these moments become more frequent and longer lasting, as with most symptoms of dementia.

> One common term you may have heard of is "sundowning." This refers to a confused state that begins in the late afternoon and lasts throughout the night.

People switching their days and nights and becoming confused about their routine (meal times, hygiene, etc.) can lead to many challenging behaviors such as confusion, aggression (protection), and anxiety. It can also cause individuals to pace and wander in agitation as they are trying to make sense of the world around them.

For caregivers at home, managing these symptoms is extremely challenging. Sleep cycles and rhythms are disrupted when a loved one has sundowner's syndrome so caregivers barely sleep as they try to ensure the person's safety overnight, and they must be awake during the day to manage usual tasks such as appointments, shopping, and cooking. This can create tremendous caregiver fatigue.

This is also a challenging symptom in nursing homes since there are usually fewer staff members available at night. Less staff makes it harder to offer personalized and timely interventions to help a person who is in distress. Unfortunately, without personalized approaches and specific training, the solution is often medication.

"Don't tell me what to do!"

You're an adult, right? You read your own mail. Go to the bank. Cook your meals. Decide when you are going to shower. Choose your own clothes. Imagine suddenly there is someone in your life telling you multiple times a day that you don't know what you are doing, what you are doing is wrong, and the person demands that you stop your behavior so he or she can take over the task. I would be furious if someone tried to boss me around in this way. Becoming angry is a reasonable reaction when we're being bullied, pushed, or forced into doing or not doing things that we know we can handle on our own.

When people don't understand what is happening around them, the natural response is to pose questions and, depending on the circumstances, to express doubt or concern. Many times, a person with dementia becomes angry, because, let's face it, wouldn't you become angry if your kids tried to tell you that you don't know how to write a check? Can you imagine if your child had the nerve to tell you that you haven't taken a shower in three weeks and that you smell? Who wouldn't fly off the handle?

I find that this is one of the most difficult symptoms for caregivers. They have the best of intentions to step in and manage something with which their loved one is struggling and are met with high levels of resistance and denial. Now, when I'm of sound mind, of course I can say that I want my kids to help me pay my bills, prepare meals, and make sure I'm groomed. Of course. If I need help, I hope that someone is there to protect me and help me.

> **With dementia, insight, decision-making, and judgment begins to disappear so our loved ones are no longer able to evaluate the risks and consequences of their decisions.**

When people have dementia, they cannot properly evaluate the risks and benefits of their choices, and they lack the insight and memory to understand that not paying the electricity bill leads to the power being disconnected. As a result, when the family highlights these issues and tries to take over, they are seen as interfering and meddling in affairs that are none of their business. Seniors already feel as if they are viewed as less capable and "old and confused." So, when a loved one steps up and verbalizes incompetence it's like pouring salt on an open wound. Most times the person doesn't remember that you've had this discussion so each time you step in to assist them it's like opening up that wound and reminding them, once again, that they aren't managing well. This just creates ongoing periods of hostility and accusations toward family members.

> **Typically, this behavior is the most challenging in the beginning to middle stages of the disease. The person still has enough awareness to know that something is not right but doesn't have the cognitive competencies to figure out what it is.**

Caregivers become frustrated and angry too because they feel their loved one should just *know* that they want the best for them. They should understand that they are looking out for them. So, the gloves come off and the fighting begins.

There are ways in which caregivers can mitigate and reduce the anger, agitation, and defensiveness of a person with dementia. If you use common sense and think about how you would want someone to help you, you'll realize that you would not want to be treated that way. Pointing out a fault and saying what's wrong, or implying someone is incapable, is never a good approach.

Think about your own life. If your husband says to you, "I've told you a thousand times, you don't know how to manage our finances and you constantly make mistakes," what would your reaction be? I know I'd be pissed! Now, let's say your husband said, "Tell me your thought process when you are creating our budget? Can you show me so I can understand what you're doing?" This could spark a calm discussion in how approaches differ; each person would be more likely to delegate and trust if they understood the process. This being said, I know that in this example these are two individuals who don't have dementia and gaps in their cognitive functioning.

I suggest you take this non-accusatory type of approach and adapt it to your loved one's abilities. In the case of a missed electricity bill you might say, "Wow, Dad. How strange you don't have electricity. Can you show me where your last statement is so we can figure this out together?" This could start a discussion in which your parent shares their steps in managing, or really not managing, their finances.

At some point you can say, "Well, I'm not sure how this happened as you do have a system in place. But let's see if we can call the company and clear things up." You know the system is not in place. You know your parent made a mistake. So what? You'll have to let go of the need to be right in almost all of these scenarios. The focus should be on minimizing your loved one feeling stupid or incompetent and reducing the number of arguments and anger. Then it's a win-win.

At some point, the conversation about your observations and concerns between you and your loved one has to happen. I know it's uncomfortable and many times can incite anger. But the longer you wait the more risk is involved. There is a greater chance of more missed payments, overpayments, being taken advantage of, and other risks. I suggest you approach your loved one when you are ready for any reaction, knowing that your intention is to protect him or her and that you are doing this out of love. It helps to remember this if your loved one gets angry.

In my opinion, honesty is important and I suggest families start with an honest discussion. But I understand that there must be a balance between mitigating risk, preserving relationships, and being honest. For example, if your father has been getting into car accidents but refuses to stop driving, what do you do? Do you take away the keys in order to protect his safety and that of others? When he forgets you took the keys away and then searches the home endlessly, do you remind him that you took them? What will this do to your relationship? Will he become so angry that he refuses to see you and now you don't have access to his home to bring him groceries, manage his medication, and keep him safe?

Or do you pull out the battery wire and pretend the car is broken and the local garage is under construction and that he will have to wait to get it fixed, hoping that in a few weeks he will just let go of his fight to drive? We all have to balance risk, safety, relationships, and honesty, and I make no judgments toward families who do what is necessary to keep their loved one safe and accessible.

The other key ingredient is compassion. Often, someone recognizes that his or her mind is not functioning as it had in the past. Fear often prevails and people go into protection mode, which for most means denial. If we don't acknowledge what's happening maybe it will just go away. Before you initiate this conversation, imagine yourself down the road experiencing the same type of symptoms. How would you want your children or spouse to approach you? Lead with that in mind.

Gently start the conversation with statements like, "Mom, I love you so much and want the best for you. I want to share some concerns I have so we can come up with a plan to figure out what's happening and find a solution. I've noticed that for the past three months you have had more difficulty organizing your bills and making payments. Have you noticed this too?" If your mom denies this, you can again tell her gently that from your perspective this isn't the case. "Mom, I appreciate that you feel that you are managing your financial responsibilities as you always had. Perhaps you are. However, for the past three months you've asked me to help you. Would you be open to pulling out your financial papers and taking me through how you organize things? Maybe there are some ways in which I can help you?"

"Mom, I already told you that"

This symptom is a real live Groundhog Day. It's a loop of exhaustion for caregivers. In my clinical work, I am used to being asked multiple times during my visits for my name and the reason why I'm there and hearing the same story again and again. But this is a time-limited thing for me as a professional. After the interview I return home to my family and, if I'm honest, find myself often repeating things to my children like "brush your teeth"...but that is completely different.

Short-term memory loss usually appears gradually, beginning with something like "I can't find my glasses" or forgetting a conversation or an appointment.

> As we age, we all notice that our memories aren't as sharp. But for most people, this is not a symptom of dementia. It may be a mild cognitive impairment that never advances and certainly does not interfere with our daily functioning.

For many people, myself included, what is commonly referred to as "a senior moment" isn't that frightening. We can usually identify that these moments come the day following a night of poor sleep or when we are overwhelmed or stressed. Panic rarely sets in. But, when a loved one asks you, "When is your dad coming home for dinner?" and your dad died two years ago, hearts sink and panic begins.

Short-term memory loss can be mild and not cause significant functioning impairments. It can cause ongoing annoyances for family members who must endure, yet again, the story of how Uncle Fred started his business, a story only entertaining to Uncle Fred himself. But again, it's not harmful or risky, particularly for someone who is organized and sets up systems and routines to ensure details aren't lost. Many people make lists and keep them in the same location in their house and create the habit of going to that list every time there is something they know they should be remembering but can't. Others set phone or watch alarms to remind them to take their medication or that Wednesday is trash day and to bring out the garbage cans. There are also paid systems, such as automatic phone calls to remind people to take medication.

For others, short-term memory loss can lead to very scary situations, like missed doses of a medication that sends somebody to the hospital, or withdrawing money and losing it, or even worse, giving it again and again to a predatory family member or "friend." It is appropriate and expected that caregivers worry about this symptom, knowing that at any moment a person can be taken advantage of and the family may not be made aware until it is too late.

When you first notice that your loved one is starting to forget events or conversations it is important to initiate a discussion. The earlier we intervene the better. There are medications available that can help to slow down the progression of the disease but are typically only effective in the earlier stages of the disease. Obviously, we don't want to miss the opportunity for early intervention.

For example, if your mom has forgotten a detail you mentioned about your work, you might say something like, "Mom, I've been noticing that you have forgotten that I got a promotion and this is something that you would remember since it is of such importance in my life. Has anyone else commented on you forgetting details lately? Is this something you've noticed about yourself?"

"My neighbor is stealing from me! Call the cops."

Imagine this. You go outside to your mailbox to collect your mail and see your neighbor across the street standing on his porch. He waves to you and says, "Hi, Ms. Erickson. How are you today?" You quickly turn and head inside, locking the door. You look outside the window and see that your neighbor is still outside seemingly looking at your door. You just know that he has been stealing your mail. You haven't received your bank statements for months, and the last time you went to the bank the balance was lower than what it is normally. Does he watch for the postal carrier to arrive so he can surreptitiously steal your mail and then take your bank account information? It must be him. After all, he is very kind to you so he must be trying to throw you off the trail. And wait! Is he friends with the bank teller? She is awfully nice to you too.

Unfortunately, for some individuals diagnosed with dementia, paranoia and delusions are part of the presenting symptoms. It is heartbreaking to watch a person be convinced that someone is trying to hurt him or take advantage of him. He is afraid, angry, and anxiety-ridden as he tries to do anything he can to prevent this "crime" from happening. Many people refuse to leave their homes or see their loved ones as their brain persuades them into believing that this would be risky. Some even turn to virtual strangers to entrust them with personal and financial information, convinced that their loved ones are out to get them… but this "friend" is the one to trust.

I have seen many caregivers who are devastated when a parent thinks they are trying to steal from them when all they have tried to do is help. Families are worried about the deterioration of a home environment or physical health when a person with paranoia or delusions often isolates himself or herself. It is very sad and often leads to a crisis in which the person may be hospitalized or forced to move into a secured setting, which of course only further amplifies the paranoia.

Quick and Easy Strategies

Here are a few easy ways to make the living environment calm and patient-friendly for someone diagnosed with dementia. Essentially, you are adjusting the environment to the person's symptoms rather than the person having to adjust to the environment.

In some residences, the staff wear pajamas in the early evening to give a visual cue that nighttime is approaching. Families could do this in the home too. Some residences have videos playing throughout the building with images of individuals brushing their teeth and climbing into bed. Again, this is a visual cue. There are more and more residences that are actually mini-villages in which the hallways and front doors are designed to resemble a neighborhood and the indoor shopping "mall" is enclosed and safe. It is made to feel like a real home, not a hospital.

Some residences have nonstop walking loops so a person who

wanders around can continue on a path and never hit a dead end. Music could be played throughout the building that reflects the era of the residents, not the staff. Staff may delegate small tasks to individuals to make them feel useful, such as folding towels or setting the table. Animals are wonderful for people young and old and can offer much needed unconditional love and affection. More recently, unique dolls that are so lifelike that I have to take a second glance are offered to residents to cuddle and speak to as if they are a baby. There are animal versions of these dolls as well. Certainly, fresh air is needed for everyone, so an enclosed outdoor area is beneficial. Some senior residences even have daycare centers within the same building since young children can be so joyful and loving and healing for us all.

There are some precautions to take in establishing a daycare center in the same building with older adults. Kids are the ultimate germ carriers and older adults are at a higher risk for health complications, so being around young children frequently all the time could pose a health threat to seniors. Being around young children who make noise and cry could be disturbing for someone who has a mild neurocognitive disorder (dementia). Sometimes people with dementia can become verbally or physically aggressive if they feel threatened or uncomfortable, and these outbursts can be unpredictable. Young children may be frightened by this behavior so it is important that everyone's participation in these types of programs is evaluated regularly.

There are so many more ideas that can easily be added to any environment to support someone with dementia. If you'd like more information on these topics you can follow me on social media or visit www.stephanieerickson.ca as I post examples of environments, strategies, etc. for family and professional caregivers to consider.

Key Take-Home Messages

At www.stephanieerickson.ca you can download toolkits to help you with the evaluation and implementation of all things aging if you are looking for further information. But here is a quick summary.

I suggest that you and your family do the following now.

1. Discuss cognitive deficits and the continuum of care required should this situation arise in your family. Explore values, fears, resources, and expectations related to housing, medical care, spiritual support, emotional support, visitations, etc.

2. Talk about what legal documents are needed, such as a Power of Attorney, Healthcare Surrogate, Living Will, and a Last Will and Testament with your family, attorney, friends, etc. Prepare them and share them with those designated on the documents.

When your parent is at home with a cognitive loss:

1. Find out who your parent's primary physician and specialists are and ask your parent that you be included in his or her file as an emergency contact. If possible, ask your parent to sign an authorization form allowing the

physician to speak with you about your parent's health.

2. Make a list of all medications and the contact information for all treating physicians to keep with you in the case of an emergency.

3. Give your name and phone number to a neighbor should he or she have any concerns about your parent's behavior.

4. Upon diagnosis (if not prior), be certain your parent prepares legal documents such as a Healthcare Proxy/ Power of Attorney/Living Will/Last Will and Testament.

When your parent is in the hospital with a cognitive illness:

1. Immediately introduce yourself to the head nurse, social worker, and physician and ask that your name be included on the emergency contact form. If your parent is able to express his or her opinion, ask him or her to inform the staff that you are to be involved in decisions and have your parent sign a document to that effect (if he or she is competent to do so).

2. Present your legal document (Healthcare POA, Healthcare Proxy, Living Will, etc.) to the care team so that your position as a care partner is established.

3. Ask for a team meeting within three days of your parent's admittance and request follow-up meetings every two weeks.

4. Insist that you be present for the discharge meeting and ask for resources about the following: housing, home care, rehabilitation, medication changes, how to identify an

emergency requiring a re-hospitalization, and resources for all of the above.

5. Upon diagnosis of a neurocognitive disorder or other health problem, ensure that your parent prepares legal documents such as a Healthcare Proxy/Power of Attorney/ Living Will/Last Will and Testament.

When your parent with a cognitive illness is in a residence:

1. Introduce yourself to the general manager, social worker, and head nurse immediately and request an admission's meeting. If your parent is able to express his or her opinion, ask him or her to inform the staff that you are to be involved in decisions and have your parent sign a document to that effect. If not, share any legal document that you have that gives you the authority to be involved.

2. Provide contact details for all family members and review the facility's emergency procedures, visitation, recreation, medication administration, and communication policies.

3. Request a follow-up meeting two weeks post-admission, and then every three to six months to ensure quality of care.

4. Every time you visit, purposefully greet the head nurse so that your ongoing presence and involvement is noted. If you visit after-hours, you can leave a note occasionally or ask to have a nurse's aide place a note in the chart noting your presence.

5. Upon diagnosis (if not prior), ensure that your parent prepares legal documents such as a Healthcare Proxy/ Power of Attorney/Living Will/Last Will and Testament.

CHAPTER 4

The Aging Heart and Soul

Why we call aging entering the "golden years" is beyond me. I have never met anyone over the age of seventy who speaks of his or her life as golden. Sure, there are wonderful things that can be occurring at this stage—grandchildren, travel, hobbies, retirement, volunteering, free time. But there are other things that come with the territory. For most, there are emerging health concerns. A change in mobility. A decrease in energy. Many also have financial concerns as they speculate if there will be enough funds to last for the lifespan and/or pay for care or housing that might be required. Grief is common, as peers become ill or die. For many, thoughts of relocation into a "safer" environment begin.

As we age, we reflect on the life we have led. We may also contemplate our (possible) suffering and wonder what we did in our lives to deserve this. Many plead with God or a Higher Power or the Universe for relief. Spiritual crises arise as we begin to feel the end of our life approaching. As we are older, we feel less useful and question what the purpose of everything is.

Loss becomes the norm as we get older. It is not only the loss of people, but the loss of our health, mobility, neighborhoods (if we have to move), our driver's license (for many), our minds (for many as well), and our purpose (since we no longer work and as discussed in the introduction, many older adults lose "value" in our society as they no longer "contribute"). We recognize that more life is behind us than in front of us and we begin to wonder if we did it right.

> **It is not surprising that many older adults suffer from depression.**

Depression and anxiety are NOT a normal part of aging, but they're not an unusual occurrence. Based on what I've seen in the struggles that families endure when trying to arrange support for an older adult who needs assistance, it's not surprising that these vulnerable groups experience depression and anxiety, as do caregivers and family, which I will address later. Mental health is at the core of who we are, how we function, and how we enjoy and embrace life. Unfortunately, there is still a stigma attached, and for older adults, I hear a lot of statements like, "Well of course she's depressed; she just moved into a residence," almost flippantly, as if because it is an anticipated reaction due to the circumstances it is therefore unnecessary to address.

> **Emotional and spiritual pain can manifest as physical pain.**

How many times has your neck hurt when you are feeling overwhelmed and stressed? When my anxiety is high, my hips hurt terribly as I'm locking all of my anxiety tight into my pelvis. Contradictory to the medical model, when we manage and address emotional and spiritual pain, our physical pain decreases. If we want to improve someone's physical health we cannot ignore their mental health.

Our Internal Self

I have included the emotional, psychological, and spiritual (soul) of aging together in one chapter. These are how I make the distinction between each. Our emotional self is made up of our feelings and how relationships and experiences impact our personality. Our psychological self is more of our thought processes, belief systems, insight, judgments, and perceptions of larger concepts. Our spiritual self is based on the meaning we attach to our experiences and how it makes us feel whole or fractured. It is the piece of us that connects with others' pain and suffering as a global community.

For example, when my dad died, I had an emotional reaction— grief, sadness, depression, and anxiety. Psychologically it made me view life differently. I understood in real time how short life is and how quickly we can lose someone we love. Spiritually, I asked myself why did this happen to my dad and what was I supposed to learn from this horrible experience. These may not be how others differentiate these three parts of who we are, but for me, this is how I see it. But the lines between each of these are blurry and fluid so I decided to lump them together to demonstrate how easily one area influences the other and impacts our overall mental health.

The Psychology of Aging

Erik Erikson, a renowned psychologist from the 1950s, espoused a very useful theory with which I agree. Developmental milestones don't just apply to children. It's not only about when we first sat up, first walked, or spoke our first words. There is a psychological and emotional development that happens throughout the lifespan. At every age we are meant to "achieve" a milestone, and if we don't our development is impaired, altered, stalled…and this will impact every subsequent stage.

As high school and university students, we learn about child development and acquire at least a basic understanding that the relationship between a baby and his caregivers is important, and without this solid bond the child will not develop in the same emotionally healthy way. We all expect that an adolescent will rebel from her parents to develop her own sense of self. We are aware, tolerant, and supportive of these processes.

Do we learn about adulthood and older adulthood in the same way? No. But are these times in our lives any less important? Not at all. Erik Erikson developed the theory of eight stages along the lifespan that explain our biggest emotional and psychological objectives at any given age. Why do I bring this up? Because when we are older, these stages, these objectives matter.

In our last stage, Integrity vs. Despair (from the age of sixty-five and older) we are reviewing our lives. We analyze and evaluate our entire lifespan, reflecting on the decisions we made and the relationships we built. We think about our successes and failures and ponder if we've wasted our shot at living life right. When we feel good about our life we feel fulfilled and satisfied. This makes it much easier to cope with the physical changes that come with aging, the health crises, and thinking about our eventual death and legacy. Aging isn't tranquil, but it can be easier when we feel like we've had a good life.

What happens to seniors who, once they reach this stage of reflection, have regrets? For example, they may feel remorse over the decisions they made, such as focusing on their career at the expense of building solid relationships with their family. How do you think a person stuck in despair manages physical pain? Emotional pain? Isolation from family because of his poor relationship with them while he built his career? As this person moves closer to the end of his life, he may be bitter, angry, resentful, and depressed.

What if a woman was often angry at her children when they were younger? She yelled at them or was even physically abusive? How do you think she feels now when her children aren't calling her or visiting her? She likely feels intense guilt about her parenting and remorse over her actions. This could lead to her reluctance to ask for assistance from her kids, or to isolate herself from others, feeling that she doesn't deserve any love at this stage in her life. This slow-downed time of a senior's life is an opportunity to process his or her regrets and remorse to help clear their mind and soul from deep historical pain. This emotional release will help them reduce physical pain and accept death as it creeps closer.

We must pay attention here. Older adults are asking themselves questions all the time. "When will I die?" "Will I be in pain?" "Will I be alone?" "Am I a burden to my family?" "What have I done to deserve this?" When we shove people into the corner and turn on the television, many of their questions are answered. "Yes, you'll be alone. No one will notice your pain. Your fear is real. You don't matter."

> **The point of this is that after we reach age sixty-five, and even more so as the years advance, we need MORE care and attention. We need family, friends, and healthcare professionals who don't find us to be a burden or an afterthought. We need to be surrounded by patient individuals who prompt discussions about our lives, encouraging and supporting us as we process and reflect and help us come to terms with our current state.**

But what do we do to that group, especially when they're closer to eighty years old? We send them off to a "facility" to live out their final days in a sterile environment staffed by a rotation of individuals who may or may not be invested in their work. (Side note: Pay attention to that word, "facility." Isn't it a word used to describe a place where manufacturing and production occurs? Doesn't this in and of itself say something about how we treat older adults?)

When I walk into a residence and see the line of wheelchairs with most of their occupants practically comatose and checked out (maybe due to medication, maybe due to a lack of stimulation), my heart breaks. These people should be discussing their life! Their experiences. Their relationships. Their adventures.

I recognize that staff may not have much time to sit down and generate an in-depth conversation, primarily due to poor staff-resident ratios. But conversation can be inserted into care and little moments. For example, as a staff member is pushing a wheelchair she can ask her resident, "Mr. Smith, I understand you love fishing. What's the biggest fish you ever caught?" For this same gentleman, the residence can provide or ask the family to bring in different fishing bait so that he can sift through them, remembering his fishing trips. There could be a fishing show on the television. It's no wonder why older adults are at risk for depression when they are left unstimulated as their lives are forgotten.

It's not only professional healthcare workers who can make greater strides in supporting and connecting with seniors. Families must make the effort too. I understand that family caregivers have competing responsibilities with work, their own families, and other things so they feel rushed and impatient. But it's important to take the time to sit quietly and listen, really listen, to their loved one's stories, even if they have heard them many times before. The connection and feeling of joy that a person feels when listened to far exceeds whatever small annoyance you may feel listening to the story again.

> **One day you will be old too and you will want someone to listen to you.**

Spoiler alert, you will actually learn so much about life by talking with your older loved ones. My perspective on what matters most has been shaped by my clients (and my parents and grandparents). Lessons and insight are a gift you will receive if you just take a minute and listen.

Older adults, especially those with health problems, need psychological support. But our system is a medical model that rarely takes into consideration the emotional and psychological health of individuals.

Recently, I was asked to assist a family in advocating for their mother who was in the healthcare system in a rehabilitation residence. They wanted her time to be extended, even though she no longer qualified, according the healthcare system's criteria. My client, an eighty-year-old woman, had fallen and broken her neck and required extensive physical rehab due to her significantly reduced mobility. For the first month after her accident the healthcare professionals continued to say that the progress the patient was making wasn't fast enough. Ultimately, they transferred her from the hospital to a long-term care nursing home, which limited her access to rehabilitation services to once a week.

What was never considered, nor offered until I became involved, was that this woman was suffering from depression, and likely PTSD because of the trauma of her fall. One day she was walking and the next she was bedbound, incontinent, unable to walk and unable to feed herself. It was obvious why she had spent the first several weeks sleeping. Her body was depleted and so was her mind. No one on the healthcare team offered to bring in a psychologist to help the woman deal with the trauma. How could her emotional and psychological functioning not be considered? I'll tell you why. Our systems focus on a medical model and rarely consider that someone's emotional state must be treated simultaneously for real healing to occur.

> **We must have a team approach in making sure that our emotional and psychological needs are met. Families should not be intimated or afraid to speak up about the mental health of their loved one and access to resources.**

Community Is Best

We are social beings and we do better as a community. Yes, there are individuals who really do prefer to be alone, but most of us crave some sort of interaction from friends, family, colleagues, neighbors, or even the clerk at the counter of a retail store. When we are left alone we wither. And for an elderly population, cognitive functioning can dip when we have no social or intellectual stimulation.

When someone stays at home, social interaction tends to fade as the years advance. Perhaps we no longer drive, or only want to drive locally. Maybe some of our friends have died and we have fewer options for social interaction. Or maybe we're on a fixed budget and paying for a gym membership or a cooking class isn't feasible. Many older adults are well versed with technology and can "Google" and locate community programs. But those who cannot are limited to the happenstance mailer or announcement that is delivered to their home. Being home alone all day is the exact opposite of what we need in our later years.

Everyone seems to live in a bubble. We aren't paying much attention to our neighbors or reaching out to find out what they need. We wave as we exit or get into our car and maybe toss out a "Hi. How ya doing?" But we really don't want the answer.

As a society, I believe we should have good neighbor programs, like the old "neighborhood watch" programs that built communities. We should view the residents on our block as extended family where everyone looks out for everyone else. It's not so hard to bring over a plate of lasagna to an elderly neighbor to ensure he has a hot meal. It takes only a minute or two to pick up a neighbor's mail each day and bring it to her door so she can avoid the stairs, which are a risk for her. How about stopping by before your trip to the local grocery store to check in to see if there is something that you can pick up? It's not that hard.

A few years ago, one of my neighbors who was in her eighties had fallen and subsequently had a hip replacement surgery. She was given a few weeks of rehabilitation and then sent home. Her son is a wonderful man who visited her often, bringing her groceries and checking in. But he couldn't be there all the time. On Thursdays I would carry her garbage cans out to the curb and back, as did another set of neighbors on our block.

In addition, three or four times a week when I was outside with my kids, supervising them playing catch or drawing with chalk on the sidewalk, I would knock on my neighbor's door and ask her if she was ready for her walk. I carried her walker down her porch stairs and assisted her stepping down. Then I would take a short walk with her to the end of the block and back to keep her walking. It took about fifteen minutes. It was great for her, and in truth, it was wonderful for me too. She told me stories about her kids growing up on our block and their years at the local pool where my family are now members. As an added benefit, my kids watched me take care of a neighbor, giving my time to another person in my community. Hopefully, they will take this memory with them into the future and do the same in their community.

Not only does this build a connection, a neighbor could see some warning signs if people aren't well, or not answering their door.

> **I suggest that you have at least two phone numbers of neighbors who live near your elderly family member so that you can check in if there is an emergency. And these neighbors should have your phone number so that they can call you should they suspect something is wrong with your loved one.**

Of course, your elderly family member should be involved in this link with neighbors—nothing should be done behind a person's back. These connections within our community will reduce the risk of depression for seniors and create a safety net in times of crisis.

We Are Not Just a Number

We make an emotional connection with every single person with whom we cross paths. Eye contact, a handshake, and a squeeze of the shoulder are small gestures that let people know that they aren't alone. You show them that all people matter and you see them. When older adults are in a residence, many go "unseen." Too often the staff I meet don't know their patients.

A few weeks ago, I arrived at a nursing home to visit a patient. This was my first visit and I wanted to introduce myself to the nurse as a professional courtesy. When I gave my name and stated the name of my client, the nurse had to look on the board to see who this person was and in which room she was. When I asked if I could have a moment of the nurse's time later to find out about how my client was functioning she said to me, "I have no idea. I don't even know who she is. You'll have to ask the other nurse. Except she's on vacation for two weeks."

Do you know how long this client had been living there? TWO MONTHS. And who was caring for this client while the other nurse was out on vacation? I understand that nurses are assigned their regular patients, but really? Someone is in your residence, under your eyes for two months and you don't know who she is? I left that residence sick to my stomach. If we don't even know who the people are who live in our work environment, do you think their emotional needs are being met?

All residences have charts. All employees are expected to read them and to know their patients. So why isn't this happening? My gut tells me it has to do with staff/patient ratios as well as scheduling that doesn't allow for time to read charts upon arrival at work. Reading charts is important as it ensures that any new interventions, symptoms, or problems are known by all staff starting their shift. At the bare minimum, residences can always have some sort of "New Protocol" board that lists essential changes in the care of which staff can be made aware quickly.

> **Psychological and emotional support doesn't always have to be so formal. In nursing homes, emotional and psychological support can be integrated into every interaction, every moment between staff and a patient, such as discussing a person's interest in art, music, or perhaps their career, as the aide is giving a bath or pushing a client in his wheelchair into the dining room.**

Earlier this year I went to another residence to visit a client. It is a very large residence with autonomous, semi-autonomous, and dependent older adults. While I waited to sign in at the lobby entrance I observed one of the receptionists speak rudely to a resident. This man was obviously confused as he was carrying a bag of laundry with him and was trying to understand what to do with it.

This receptionist, using a raised and curt tone, told him that it wasn't her problem to solve and to make his way down the hallway. He continued to ask questions, not quite understanding these instructions, and she continued to repeatedly speak to him aggressively. I couldn't believe that a receptionist at a senior home could be so rude and lax. When she was hired, wasn't she told that there may be a confused patient who asks for help? Was she given any training? And where was this woman's compassion?

This brief moment could have been so different for this man. He could have been understood, helped, and made to feel important and that his problem was important. The receptionist could have spoken to him gently and slowly, and if necessary, call a nurse for assistance. Instead, he was treated as an inconvenience and not as someone who has feelings and a lifetime of experience behind him that should be respected.

We can also have wonderful moments worked into daily care routines. A personalized greeting from a nurse's aide to her patient like, "Hey, Mr. Bailey. What happened yesterday in the world? I saw you reading the paper." And need I say that each individual should be greeted by their name and not "honey"? (OMG, that drives me bonkers.)

I will say that I have seen some lovely interactions between staff and patients. Jokes being made followed by mutual laughter. Sweet conversations in which grandchildren and their accomplishments are being discussed. But mostly I see clients being treated like a package being moved around as one would move a box, or fed indifferently while the staff gaze off, scooping and feeding, scooping and feeding. Staffing is minimal and those who are present are busy trying to get all of the tasks done and don't have time for small talk. With high care demands and chronic understaffing, it's a recipe for disaster.

But I won't accept it. I don't believe that even if you have too many patients, you cannot find a moment during the time you're there delivering care to be kind. It takes time to get someone dressed, or assist with a bath. There are always moments in which you can ask people about their family and their accomplishments and use that information in each intervention to build a relationship and to let patients know that their life matters. What they have to say is important and valuable.

The team must ensure that emotional support, in a formal or informal way, is being provided in the same way physical care is. One is not more important than the other. The team must create opportunities for older adults to achieve integrity in the psychological stage in which they are. If your mother always wore lipstick, then make sure her team knows this. It doesn't matter if she is confused and unaware; that was something that was important to her and should continue to be important. We feel cared for and loved when details are paid attention to, and this should not change as we age.

Prompting Life Review

As I discussed above, as we get older we spend more and more time reflecting on our life, re-playing positive and negative memories in our mind, and coming to terms with the life we led. Families and care teams can work together to ensure that older adults are given the opportunity to express themselves.

Families can bring in photo albums and hang pictures to encourage life review. Families can even make notes near these photos for the staff such as "Ask my dad about his travels to Australia" or "Ask my mom about her love of cooking." This can prompt and encourage the staff to make a personal connection and bond.

Families should make an effort to show the same interest toward the staff, using their names and learning something about their lives. Of course, showing appreciation and thanks can go a long way in creating a mutually respectful relationship.

> **Whether someone is in a long-term residence or not, we can create opportunities for life review. It should be a multi-generational activity, and technology is an excellent way to get the entire family involved.**

I suggest using a phone and filming an "interview" between family members. Ask your aging relative about his life and record it. Dig through boxes of photos and memorabilia and record your relative recounting the story surrounding that photo or item. Compile family recipes and cook them together. Ask the younger generation to do the filming and to edit together a short family movie. You can also scan all of the old photos, and take pictures of memorabilia and ask the younger generation to make an online photo book (which can be printed and given to the older adult). These are treasures for all family members and future generations to cherish.

Feeding the Soul

How do you feed your soul? Do you go to church? Synagogue? A mosque? Do you pray at home alone? Do you meditate to the universe for guidance and support? Or maybe you are agnostic and are unsure of what's out there. Or you are atheist and don't believe there is anything or anyone that has created or takes care of the world. That's okay. This is not about believing in a "God" or any other power.

Feeding your soul is about understanding what it is that makes you feel at peace and gives you some time to reflect. For example, I love the beach. I'm crazy for it. Whenever I dig my toes into warm sand, feel the breeze grazing my skin, hear the pounding of the ocean and kids laughing, and smell the salt in the air, I am at peace. I feel calm. Grounded. I get the world in those moments and feel tranquility. The beach feeds my soul.

So, since I am who I am, I have already explained this to my husband and kids. Should something happen to me (now, when I'm still youngish or in my older years) and I cannot get out, bring the beach to me. Fill a bucket with sand and put my feet in it. Mix up water and salt and let me smell it. Play the sounds of the ocean on an iPad for me. This is spiritual care.

Of course, spiritual care can also be provided in more traditional ways. I was surprised recently when a daughter told me that her mother was very involved in her church and was very religiously grounded. Now, her mother in an Alzheimer's unit at a residence, and although there was a service once a week, that was the only support she was getting. I asked the daughter if she had contacted her mother's church to see if one of the members could make some visits and read scripture. This daughter smiled and said, "I never thought of that. Yes, I'll ask." It didn't matter that this woman who had Alzheimer's disease did or didn't understand the words read to her; she would connect with the feeling of spirit and religion, community and prayer.

> **In my opinion EVERY residence should employ a full-time chaplain who can spend time with every resident and provide spiritual support, even in the form of a bucket of sand.**

Woof!

We are missing the mark when it comes to the healing power of animals. Studies show how animals impact physical health with the reduction of blood pressure, improvement of cardiovascular health, and releasing endorphins, which helps to elevate mood. Animals are also nonjudgmental. They don't care if you are in a wheelchair. They don't care if you have an illness or are confused. They provide unconditional love and companionship and can lift anyone's mood with a tail wag and a cuddle. Animals can also be used in specific therapeutic ways, such as for those who suffer from anxiety or depression.

I am happy to see that more residences are introducing animal-assisted therapy and companionship on a regular basis. There are even some private residences (non-government) that have a dog or cat on site 24/7. I believe that animals should be a part of any team. Of course, if a person hates animals this doesn't make sense, but for many individuals this is an excellent way to provide emotional support.

Dogs integrated into a senior's environment is an addition that can provide immediate and lasting benefits. It will take commitment from the residence to ensure the dog is walked, bathed, and fed, so there will be some staff time that must be allotted to care for the dog. There is also the added expense of the occasional veterinary visit or annual rabies shot. At a few residences in which I've visited, a staff member brings their own personal dog to work daily. This way, there is no extra expense for the dog and the staff member can take it on a walk a few times during the day.

Cats are an easier implementation. They are not typically social or cuddly, but there are some cats out there that love to sit in a senior's lap for hours on end. Cats are very low maintenance for staff too. Some residences allow their clients to bring their own animals with them when they move in, and I find this magical for the client and the rest of the residents. Any way it can be done, the benefit of having dogs or cats in a senior's environment far exceeds the commitment from the residents or staff.

Another option are robotic dogs and cats, which I admit horrified me when they were first introduced. I questioned why real animals were not being used and hypothesized it was likely a cost issue and a time investment for staff who would need to take time away from residents to take the dog on a walk. However, this month while visiting a client I observed a patient (not mine) sitting with a robotic cat in her lap. Each time she scratched its neck it purred and batted its eyes and the patient's eyes lit up in delight. She was whispering loving words to this "cat" for the entire hour I was there. On my way out, my client stopped next to this woman and began to pet the cat as well, calling me over to show me how beautiful he was. So, I guess I'm sold. First choice are real live animals, but these robotic animals seem to be providing comfort so they should be considered helpful as well.

Music to My Ears

Every time I hear "We Are Family" from Sister Sledge I am transported to high school when me and my girlfriends sang and danced to this song as a tribute to one another. When I hear "Could This Be Love" from Bob Marley I am dancing at Club Med with a guy I just met, as we made googly eyes at each other, and whom I married three years later.

My father-in-law, even during the late stages of his dementia, could sing "*La feuille d'érable*," word for word with perfect tone and vibrato. It was beautiful to hear. (Side note: We have it recorded too so that even now that he is deceased, we have his lovely voice with us.) Music is magical. It sparks memories. It can get us pumped up for a challenge. It can calm us down when we are spiraling. Music sets the mood for any occasion.

To me this is one of the easiest interventions that can be provided to anyone at any time. Unfortunately, I find the television replaces music more often. Residences, homes, hospitals, and rehabilitation facilities can all be equipped with individual sound systems that anyone can just plug an iPod or iPad or computer into and voila, we have our own personal playlist. In my opinion, healthcare institutions (institutions—I hate that word too, by the way) can ask families to provide a playlist and music can be playing around the clock to help a person relax, to stimulate memories, to prompt conversations with others, and to bring joy.

While an expensive proposition, the impact on the bottom line would be very positive. Individuals would feel better or have less pain physically and emotionally. Music playing throughout the residence would change the mood of the staff, who will in turn provide better care. I am baffled that residences are either silent or have the sound of the blaring television.

Music can also stimulate physical exercise. Residences who have activity coordinators use music and dancing to engage individuals and to get them moving. Even for people who are wheelchair or bed bound, many still have the ability to clap their hands and tap their feet to the music. I love it when I'm visiting a client and I hear singing coming from the activity room. It tells me that in that moment at least, a team member is creating a feeling of joy for the residents.

Another way to integrate music would be to involve the community. Local churches or other religious institutions, community choirs, community theater groups, veterans groups, seniors groups, daycares, or schools (especially during the holidays) are simple and free options to bring music into a residence. If there is a recreational therapist (discussed further in the Team Caregiver chapter), he or she could make these links and keep an ongoing rotation of visitors. If not, a staff person could take a few hours a month to do some outreach and set a schedule.

See, Touch, Smell, Taste

Music is a great way to bring back memories. There are other ways too. All of us have done some activity in our life that involved a "thing." Perhaps we enjoyed cooking and used spices. Maybe we liked working on cars and fixing things around the house. Maybe we sewed our children's clothes. These memories can be elicited through objects and experiences.

If your dad loved to cook, create a spice box and sit with him (and film it for the family) and have him smell each spice and recount a recipe that he loved to make, or a meal that his mother made for him as a boy. If your mom sewed, how about presenting her with different materials from silk to cotton to wool and have her describe items that she made. If she still has fine motor skill ability, why not sew or knit now? How about just rolling up a ball of yarn to stimulate a remote task that she used to do. Tools are a bit trickier because there are some dangers if people have cognitive problems. But there are products that have visuals of tools, or even non-dangerous toolkits for someone to use.

There are many, many ways in which we can stimulate the mind, prompt life review, and give meaning to the day through tactile ways. I believe that this investment by a hospital or residence would prove cost-effective because the individual would be stimulated and distracted and their overall mental health would improve.

> Our mental health is vital as we age. We must be given opportunities to reflect on our life and to give meaning to our current circumstances, and a team can make it happen creatively.

Out of the Box

The essential thing to remember about our heart and soul is that they need nourishment. We are living beings who need to connect with others and the deep parts within us. Be creative when thinking about what you could do to inspire reflection.

For example, I heard about one residence that had a beautiful outdoor garden, so they started renting it out for weddings. A few times a year, the residents would gather outside and watch a bride walk down the aisle to meet her groom. I am sure their hearts were filled as they were thrown back in time to their own wedding. In more autonomous settings some of the residents could be involved in setting up or decorating.

Another idea, if appropriate for the setting, is to throw a birthday party for one of the resident's grandchildren. Why not? Get a cake. Balloons. Play children's music. Again, the residents can sit by and watch a few kids play and dance and excitedly open gifts. This would also sensitize these children to the world of seniors and make it less scary. This could go a long way to shift the way we think about older adults and how so many cast them out.

CHAPTER 5

The Aging Body

Oof. Ugh. Ow. How many of you reading this recognize these sounds as ones that you make each time you stand up or sit down?

Last summer I played football on the beach with my son during our yearly trip to California. About six days into the trip I twisted my ankle while trying to catch one of his passes. Twelve months have passed and I still feel it in my ankle. I bet my ankle will remember that day for the rest of my life! If I had been twenty when I twisted it, the memory would likely be long gone as the healing would have been quick and easy.

I'm already feeling time passing in my joints and muscles. Despite working out daily, I feel the reduction in my strength. I see how my flexibility has changed. I always have some chronic ache or pain somewhere. In my mind, I still see myself as a twenty-five-year-old and think I should be able to tackle any physical challenge facing me. But that's just not the reality.

This is a problem. Our bodies age faster than our minds and we don't want to believe it. "But I'm twenty!" my mind shouts while my body disagrees and orders me to hold on to the handrail as I walk down the stairs. And even though I'm only fifty, I look carefully where I walk. I think about having both feet flat on the floor and bending my knees as I pick something up.

I am so scared of getting hurt, mostly because I know it will take months to heal and it is unlikely it would be a full-fledged recovery. I also know that two of the key factors to aging well are mobility and strength. If I'm injured, I cannot exercise as much as I do now and my aging will be hastened.

The Damn Mirror

Do you recognize yourself when you look in the mirror? Are you surprised to see that you look older than you feel? Look down at your hands. Are your veins more visible through increasingly transparent skin? Now imagine being eighty-five but feeling like you are forty and seeing the wrinkles and loose skin every time you look in the mirror. And what about your body? Is it just as tight and fit as when you were younger? Or are you a bit rounder? A bit looser? I know I am.

As I was planning my fiftieth birthday party, I was putting together a digital photo collage to project on my television during the party. For several days I poured through photos from my childhood and early adult years and scanned them into my computer.

I could not believe my eyes. When I looked at photos of me from my twenties I was stunned. It doesn't even seem like I'm the same person! My curly hair and blue eyes are the giveaway, but I was so slim and didn't have any gray hair and there were no wrinkles on my face. I long for that body and clear face. (Side note: I wish I would have celebrated how I looked during those years instead of comparing myself to others and being riddled with self-hatred. But that is a story for another day and book.)

> **It may sound shallow, but we cannot underestimate the impact of how our looks change and how this impacts how we feel about ourselves.**

The physical part of aging has many levels, and how we look is one of them. We look older, and for the majority of us we don't like what we see. The changes are slow and subtle and we don't notice them from day to day, but then...bam! One day it looks like we have aged by ten years overnight. There is absolutely nothing we can do about these changes except roll with them and find ways to love or make peace with our skin evolution.

So, if there is nothing we can do to reverse physical aging, why bring it up? Because it's hard for older people to manage these changes emotionally, and I think we are not sensitive enough to this. We are quick to say, "Oh no, you're beautiful. I don't see the changes at all." While this comment is well intended, it doesn't allow for a person to process what she sees and come to terms with it.

> **Part of aging is processing. We all need to process things to get to a place in which we can manage the discomfort, whether it's about aging or other issues we're facing.**

Particularly with aging, acknowledging that changes to our looks and bodies are in fact happening, and that this is hard, helps us to make peace with it.

In this same vein, we must help the people we care for present themselves to the world as they had when they were younger. This means different things to different people. My mother-in-law, who is ninety-one, never leaves the house without her hair beautifully done, her lipstick on, her jewelry in place, and her pocketbook on her arm. This has been her pattern for her entire life and it makes her feel like "her."

If she is ever in a situation in which she can no longer do this for herself, or if she develops a neurocognitive disorder and doesn't remember that this was a priority, I will make sure that she continues to be groomed and primed for an outing, even if she is going nowhere. Respecting someone's physical presence should never change, regardless of other health concerns. I've already coached my daughter to make sure that I never have any long black hairs growing out of my chin if my eyesight fails and I can't find them myself!

When I visit nursing homes, this is something that, to me, is a dead giveaway about whether the staff is paying attention and actually seeing the person as who he or she is now and was in the past. It drives me mad when I see photos of my client splattered around his room showing him dressed to the nines in a coat and tie, standing straight and confident, filled with pride. Then, in front of me, I see a man with his hair standing on end wearing sweat pants and a T-shirt stained with jam from the morning's breakfast. I understand that staff is pressed for time, but come on! If this person has always taken pride in his looks and hygiene, I don't care what his current state of mind is. Help him do the same now. And yes, there are adapted clothes that have button-up shirts and slacks. (What are adapted clothes? Adapted clothes make dressing and undressing easier for individuals how have a reduced range of motion or difficulty manipulating zippers and buttons. Residences may request that adaptive clothing is provided to make it easier for staff to assist their clients.)

**Our physical presentation to the world,
no matter what our state of mind, matters.**

Laughter Heals

"Oy vey," I often say under my breath as I'm trying to maneuver myself around our home. I creak and crack all the time, but I'm still heavily involved with my personal passion, the flying trapeze. I "fly" (train) twice a week and it is very strenuous on the body and takes great strength and flexibility.

Seven years ago, when I started flying, I stretched a bit before taking my first swing, which is the base of everything we do in trapeze. We must have a strong, tight, and high swing to execute tricks. A few years ago, I started to do a "granny swing" (which is what I named it) in which I just hang on the bar, allowing my body to stretch and warm up before adding any force to a swing because my body could no longer handle jumping into a full swing. You know what? Now I need two granny swings.

One of the ways my flying team and I cope with the ever-challenging physical changes that impact our ability to fly is to laugh. This is why these swings are called "granny swings." And even that has morphed into other laughable swing names. Now, I need two "granny swings" followed by a "baby swing," which means a very low-energy swing to get my joints awake, followed by an "adolescent swing," which means I can put a bit more power into it (and I usually complain while I'm swinging, as any normal adolescent would do), followed by, finally, a "real swing." My team and I crack up how over the past several years our warm-up has become so long that the training is practically over before we even begin our tricks. We often joke that one day, we should just install a lift from the ground to the platform because sometimes just climbing the ladder is exhausting.

Humor is a wonderful way to cope with the changes in our body. Laughter in and of itself has wonderful health benefits such as stimulating organs, activating a stress response, and releasing tension. Try sharing a laugh with a peer and you'll find that the comradery of facing aging lightly goes a long way in preserving our mental health.

Those Creaking Bones

Our bodies age. Over time, strength is lost. Mobility is reduced. Flexibility fades. It is the reality of getting older. Sure, we can and should exercise daily, incorporate strength training (especially in our legs to put the odds on our side that we won't end up in a wheelchair), and keep up with cardio to keep our heart healthy. All of these things work, and absolutely we should never stop moving.

The reality is that our body gets older. Period. This leads to anger and frustration when our body disobeys what our mind so clearly orders.

I can see the frustration in my grandma's face when at ninety-seven years old, she has to use a walker. She was someone who used to walk several miles a day until she was about eighty-eight. Then she worked out less strenuously on a treadmill as her back began to fail her. She can no longer exercise due to debilitating back pain and reduced mobility. Now, she uses a walker and struggles at times to transfer from a chair to a standing position. I know. From an outsider's point of view, they're likely to think, "Hooray! You're still walking at ninety-seven!" But for my grandma, her mind doesn't match her body. She cannot accept these changes and it pains her to be "slow," to need extra time, and to say no to activities and outings due to physical limitations.

We must validate the frustration and anger individuals feel when their mobility is reduced. Be patient when people need more time. It's up to you to make the adjustments to your schedule to allow for additional time in and out of the house and car. Do not exclude someone because it is too much work for you, if at all possible. Instead, make the adjustments on your end to make it work.

Imagine yourself at ninety, sitting at home, knowing your family is out celebrating or doing something wonderful and you were left behind. Imagine sitting in a chair, watching the world go by, and not being able to jump up and engage. It doesn't feel good. Be compassionate and include your loved ones as much as you can.

Illness

If you look at aging in a purely statistical sense, the older we get, the more likely we are to become ill. It makes sense. Our organs, bones, muscles, and brain all diminish with years of wear and tear. Unless we have had a serious illness as a child or a young adult, or know someone who has survived one, we tend to take our health for granted when we are young. But as we get older we begin to see our contemporaries face illness, and this sends us into moments of self-reflection, often followed by worry, as to what will happen to us.

If I'm honest, I think about illness a lot. It's likely because I'm faced with it every day in my work setting and I see what it does to individuals and families. The older I get, the more I worry. I've mentioned both my mother-in-law and my grandma in this chapter, but I can add my mom and many aunts and uncles to those who I see worry. They all talk about how hard things are as they are getting older, including watching their friends become ill. They are worried about their own health. Routine bloodwork doesn't feel so routine anymore because at any moment an unexpected result can pop up and cause them to worry about the test results.

Most of the time when we hear aging loved ones talk about their concerns about going to see their doctor for a follow-up, or we worry that a relative seems to be a "hypochondriac" and wants to go to the hospital or doctor for every sniffle, we tend to minimize their concerns. We may react that way with good intentions. We don't want our loved ones to worry. We want them to feel safe and secure. But, jumping in and saying "Don't worry, everything will be fine" is not always a good thing.

Discussing illness doesn't make it happen. Open conversations allow individuals to voice their fears and wishes and be comforted knowing their needs will be met and that they are not alone.

In addition to helping people feel positive about their health, I think we must also acknowledge their fears and normalize them. When everyone around them is getting sick and dying, who are we to pretend that this isn't their reality? When your loved one says, "I'm scared of getting the results today," we can answer, "Yes I get that. It's scary not knowing." Then we follow that up with, "I'll be there with you. I'm sure everything is fine, but if it's not, I'm here." That small twist of a response can help others feel reassured that they are not in this aging thing alone.

The Big Adieu

Yes, you will die one day. Brutal and direct, I know.

Why do I just jump right in and say this? Because we are a death-phobic society and this phobia morphs into avoidance. You know what avoidance brings? Loneliness and isolation. Do you want to die alone? I doubt it.

Our healthcare systems are the kings of death avoidance. Doctors don't consistently tell their patients the truth about a prognosis, which can sway a person to pursue painful treatments and interventions that can lead to the person spending his or her last days in pain and stuck in the hospital. Healthcare professionals often delay referring patients to the few palliative care centers available in any given city because it's just too hard to deliver the news that things are not getting better.

Talking about dying is hard for our society. Most people would rather avoid the discussions altogether than to allow someone else to be involved in designing the way the person will approach his or her death by choosing which interventions, treatments, and environment is right for him or her. Also, because healthcare professionals see "healing" in a physical sense only, they neglect to consider that there are opportunities for emotional and spiritual healing by giving people time to prepare for their death. Most people die in a hospital with tubes, wires, and the loud noises and busyness of staff surrounding them. Hospitals are the opposite of a peaceful setting, which makes it nearly impossible to live out your last days encircled by family, offered pain management, and with gentle staff tending to your soul, spirit, and body.

This creates a persistent anxiety that most people can't seem to shake. As we get older, it is normal to think about what will lead to our death. Will it be a chronic illness? An accident? A sudden heart attack? Will you die alone and in pain? Most family members don't want to discuss these things with their aging relative because it seems morbid. Since we are a death-phobic society we do all we can to avoid discussing it. But guess what? We will all die.

Pretending it won't happen and not allowing ourselves and others to process our fears and anxieties about it doesn't stop it from happening. In fact, in many ways it makes our fears the reality. If we are able to actually talk about death openly, I believe our systems will follow. Or maybe it's the opposite; our systems need to go first.

We must discuss death if we are to minimize our fears and create supportive and pain-free endings that meet our spiritual, emotional, and physical needs.

I worked as a palliative care social worker for several years. I visited terminally ill patients and their families in their own homes and in "institutions." What never stopped surprising me was that my patients were sent to "palliative care" and I would guess at least 50 percent had no idea that they had a terminal illness. It wasn't that they were "in denial." The families confirmed that the doctor never told them, or they had decided not to share this fact with their loved ones.

What? Really? This is so unfair. Unjust. Unethical. If you are not made aware that your illness is terminal, how can you spend your last days reviewing your life? Coming to terms with your mistakes? Asking for forgiveness? Reconnecting with those lost to you? Or say a goodbye that is meaningful for you and for those left behind?

My dad died of a sudden and massive heart attack. I regret the conversation we had the night before and wish I would have had the chance to tell him I love him one more time. I have to live with this regret. Fortunately, we had a good relationship so I am not riddled with guilt about how things were left unsaid or that our relationship had not been mended. But this is not the story for everyone.

Many people have complicated relationships with friends and family and we spend years angry, resentful, and bitter, allowing time to pass without healing. Aside from a situation like the one

I had with my dad, many times we know we are dying. We have a terminal illness, or we can just "tell" that we are not doing well and our time is becoming more limited. Or, we are simply getting older and know that death is looming.

> It may sound odd, but dying or the fear of an impending death can be an opportunity to make things right.

Encouraging each other to discuss death can open up many opportunities to repair what is broken. We can explain our reasons behind actions we took, decisions we made, and things we said. We can apologize, take responsibility, or express remorse. These are very important things that must happen as we get older. Releasing our heartaches and mistakes is important at any age, but it is paramount to achieving some kind of peace before our death.

This is not just a benefit for the patient. It helps the bereaved too. Questions are answered. Resentments are let go. Connections are made or strengthened. At the very minimum, it doesn't leave the bereaved wondering for years about what could have been.

There is something called complicated grief, which is when a bereaved person begins to become "functionally impaired" six months after the person's death. This would be something like significant anxiety and depression, an inability to return to work, etc. When open conversations occur between families prior to someone's death, the bereaved are less likely to experience complicated grief down the road.

In the palliative care world we talk about "emotional pain" or "spiritual pain." While this does apply to life in general, the term is used regularly in palliative care. Sometimes, the pain that appears in our bodies is not from cancer, a heart attack, or surgery. The pain is our unexpressed emotions. Our fears, shame, anger, and sadness can get locked into our very fibers and cause physical pain. Usually there is no pain management that can numb that pain. By having the opportunity to face our death, we are allowing our own bodies the chance to experience a pain-reduced death. Isn't this what we all want?

Another important part of the dying process is making our wishes known. Do we want all necessary measures to keep us alive? I'm sure you've heard the terms DNR (do not resuscitate), tube feeding, etc. When we envision our impending death, as you can at this very moment even if "impending" for you is thirty years away, we can put our wishes in writing. Only positive things come out of having your wishes clearly outlined and understood by your loved ones.

(Read Chapter Six: The Aging Pocketbook for more discussion on the importance of legal documents.)

Death can be scary. Most unknowns are. But if we feel good about the life we have led and the relationships we have built, it makes it a bit easier to face.

Inside

Even as our aging loved one's exterior changes and loses its shine, the soul, the spirit, the "being" does not fade. We always have something to offer to those around us. Let's not allow a "system" built on a disease and an interventionist model trick us into believing that a senior no longer has value. Remember that a person's experiences are alive and well inside the mind, and when given the opportunity, they are ready to be shared with the world.

CHAPTER 6

The Aging Pocketbook

"I've already put out $20,000 of my own money to prevent my parents from falling into bankruptcy. I'm not sure how much more I can do."

"My mom paid taxes her entire life and this is where she ends up? No help from the government and stuck in a crappy facility with no services?"

"Insurance only covers so much. How am I going to pay for the rehab my mom needs? I don't want her stuck in a wheelchair for the rest of her life."

We spend most of our adult years working. We drag ourselves out of bed, rush our kids off to school, and grind away to make ends meet and to save for our "golden years." Once the kids move out of the home and paying for their university years are over, we keep on working to build our nest egg so that when retirement arrives we are ready to travel the world now that we are mortgage and debt free. Maybe we'll even have enough left over to give to our children when we're gone. Well, guess what? For most of us that is far from reality.

Many of the older adults I know are struggling. All of their financial security is wrapped up in their home, if they were fortunate enough to own one in the first place. Their savings are limited and they are so concerned about having enough that they are resistant to spend on anything. I understand.

As we get older, our physical and health needs increase and we must have a way to meet those needs. Most of the time, money is the way to get what we need.

Depending on where older adults live, geographically speaking, some have more resources available to them because the government supplements care or provides it, such as in Canada. In other parts of the world, like the U.S., only the poor are eligible for governmental support. The qualification level is so low that many who are truly struggling don't receive assistance.

Even in countries in which you can get governmental support, in some way or another, it is never enough. This is true in Canada, the U.S., and other countries.

Although I live in Montreal now, I worked in the U.S. for the first decade of my social work career. Long-term care residences in both countries lack sufficient resources and staff to deliver good, consistent quality care. Those that provide "good" care, in my opinion, are mostly sub-standard if you consider what we all really need.

Yes, you can get a bath. Someone will prepare a meal. Your

medication will be delivered to you. But if you need spiritual support, you have to wait for the monthly service because spiritual care couldn't possibly be needed daily. You need help walking to the bathroom? Well, pull this cord and wait. And wait. And wait. We'll try to get to you before you have an accident.

Are you struggling with the loss of your husband? "Oh, I'm so sorry." But no, we don't have any psychological support. Sure, we have activities, as long as you can get there on your own, and participate autonomously and are interested in hitting a balloon with a racket. Again.

I sound jaded. I know. I am. I don't enjoy feeling disheartened about the healthcare system, but based on my daily interactions with families, residences, and healthcare professionals, I just can't seem to help myself.

> **If you want to have care and support that takes care of your mind, body, and soul, you'll have to pay for it. That is the unfortunate bottom line of getting old.**

The Memory Box: Housing

I want to stay in my home forever. I love my house. My kids are growing up here. I can see them as babies crawling on the floor. I remember where I sat to read to them before bed. I can hear the door slamming as they ran in and out of the house playing outside on a summer day. I know which stair creaks as I walk on it. Nothing beats the comfort of my own bed. My home feels safe, comfortable, and predictable.

At some point, I know intellectually that this home may become too much for me. There is so much to manage in a home such as snow removal, lawn care, broken faucets, a leaky roof, etc. The laundry machine is in the basement. The bathrooms are on the second floor. I'm a social worker for seniors. Of course, I know all about the dangers of stairs. But how could I ever leave?

My heart breaks when I work with seniors who are moving. More often than not, the move comes at the most unpredictable and inconvenient time. It is usually a crisis that precipitates the move. Someone falls. There is a death and the surviving spouse has dementia but there is nobody to care for her. Or the neglect of the leaking roof just turned into a flood.

No matter what the circumstance, leaving one's home is hard. Painful. Overwhelming. We must support an older adult who is making this change.

Since most seniors want to stay in their home, there are things that can be done to keep a person safe. Outfitting a home with safety mechanisms is one way to do it. Equipment such as raised toilet seats and grab bars in the bathroom and other high-risk locations can be installed. There are also alarm systems, sensors, and cameras that can be used to monitor our loved ones and others who are working in their home. You should consider privacy laws and consent to being filmed before installing a camera or sensors, but they are worth looking into for many people. These are what I call quick fixes; they require limited financial investment and can be executed rather quickly.

But there are other things that may be necessary and can be very costly. For example, maybe a bathroom or extra bedroom needs to be fully adapted or even built on the ground floor. Perhaps the stairway outside leading into the house needs to become a ramp. For some, installing a stair lift is the solution. These options are doable. But they are expensive. There are some interesting things that can be done to generate funds to outfit a home, such as reverse mortgages, but this is not the right option for everyone and please consult a financial advisor before making this decision.

If an older adult chooses this option, who is going to do the research to determine the exact adaptations needed or which stair lift is appropriate for that person? Who is going to arrange for the construction or installation? The adult children. Yep, the kids are usually brought in not only for reinforcements but to become the superintendent on the job. Let's keep in mind that most of these kids are already working. They're probably in a suit and tie by day, and in the evening out comes the hard hat and clipboard.

After doing a cost analysis, some people may decide that moving into a retirement residence, or an assisted residence, or even a full-care residence is the better option. Again, it will be the adult children who will do the research to locate, visit, and choose (hopefully *with* their parents and not in place of) the best residence into which to move. For many, the research and visits happen during the workday, which places additional stressors on the family as work piles up on their desk while they are busy helping their parent.

Residences are incredibly expensive. In some systems, like Canada's, public residences are subsidized and there is a cap amount on the fees. However, in many cases you are at the mercy of the system and its public employees to determine what kind of care you need and where you are going to live, even if it is far from your community and family. You have to go where there is a "bed," regardless of where it is in or whether the time frame works for you. Once the bed becomes available you have to commit and move. It's ready. You go.

In the U.S. if you're poor, well there is a place for you. Medicare will cover the cost of the nursing home, but this benefit really covers very little and mostly when it's related to short-term stays for rehabilitation and post-hospital care, not for long-term stays. Most Americans are under the misconception that Medicare pays for a nursing home, but it doesn't. If you fall below the poverty level, Medicaid kicks in. So many Americans are not considered "poor," even though in reality they are barely making it day to day. This so-called "lower class" and working poor will not be able to afford private care. So, what happens? Who cares for them?

In the U.S. and in Canada, private residences are very, very costly. We're talking, on average for a private room, between $4,000 and $8,500 a month in the U.S. and *at least* $4,000 on average in Canada. I don't know about you, but I don't have an extra $50,000 to $100,000 lying around.

In a private, non-governmental residence you will get some additional services, and the look and feel of the residence may resemble a hotel, but in the end, if you need physiotherapy, that's extra. If you want to see a psychologist weekly? You're paying out of pocket. Do you want someone to visit your father a few hours a day for some one-on-one companionship so you can work? What will that cost you? There are some free or low-cost community resources that can be brought into residences to supplement care, but it's often not enough. So, if there is anything extra you need, guess where it comes from? You got it. Your own pocketbook.

Now, if all of your parents' capital is wrapped up in their home, the home will have to be sold for them to move. But what if your dad needs care but your mother is fully capable? Does she have to leave their home to pay for her husband's care? If the two of them move, can they be in the same residence or will they be split apart? Talk about losses on top of losses.

Of course, there is the cost of moving, the stress of packing and downsizing, and setting up the new home. I find the biggest hurdle is the emotional stress that comes with this change. Imagine if tomorrow you're in an accident and are hospitalized. After surgery and rehab you are still not able to care for yourself and have to move into a residence. You never return home.

How does that feel? What if after 50 years of marriage you have to face the truth that you can no longer care for your ailing spouse and you and she must be separated? Because you can no longer drive, you know you are relying on your adult children and their busy lives to arrange for visits with your wife. This is crushing for couples and families, and in my opinion it is inhumane to force individuals to separate. It creates emotional and psychological pain—which can lead to physical pain and health problems—and this approach is the opposite of feeding our soul.

> **When older adults move from their homes it's not just a physical change. There is a deep and wide emotional component that accompanies them.**

Our homes are loaded with not only things but with *memories*. Each photo on the mantel, each trinket on the armoire, represents a memory, a relationship, an event. It is almost impossible thinking about parting with these objects. If we are lucky to have someone in our family take it, well at least the memory lives on. But if we are forced to throw something out, literally in the garbage, does the memory go with it?

I suggest that when moving from a home, families turn the experience into a project—a walk down memory lane that ends with a physical result and a legacy to share with future generations. As I discussed in Chapter Four, we can create memory books and videos as a way to process loss, facilitate life review, and come to terms with the changes before us.

Enlist grandchildren to film their grandparents talking about the history and memory behind important objects. Ask Grandma to make her famous cookies while filming her and write down the recipe. Compile multiple recipes and turn them into a family cookbook, which can be made with a computer or an online program. Edit these videos together for a family movie to be shown to multiple generations. Scan old photos and create an album with an online platform. You can even add text about the history behind that photo.

> **A home is so much more than four walls and a roof. It's filled with memories and feelings that are hard to leave behind. Be creative and take them with you.**

Once an older adult arrives at his or her new home, there are opportunities to make it special. Families can load the walls with paintings and photos and bring in furniture from the old home. Some choose to "fresh-start it" and buy all new furniture and bedding. Some residences have guidelines about what you can and cannot bring as well. For example, many insist on a hospital bed so someone who has spent the last 70 years in a king bed has to adjust to a single bed (which can feel infantilizing). Rooms in residences are often bare and sterile, and it is up to the families to create a cozy environment. This costs money and takes time.

In many residences, especially those that offer care, privacy is lost. Nurses don't always knock on a door before entering, and rarely do I hear permission being asked to enter. This boggles my mind. Someone wouldn't just walk into my home uninvited. Why should this be different in a residence? Do not feel bad reminding staff they should ask permission before entering a resident's room.

Some individuals share a room, especially since it is less expensive, so any privacy an older adult may crave is gone. There are benefits to having a roommate, however. Isolation is reduced, companionship and social interaction are now easier, and there is twice the chance that you can get assistance from staff.

Additional costs in residences can be utilities, a television or phone, extra chairs for visitors, maybe a small refrigerator in the room, and personal items, etc. Most of the time you must pay for grooming (haircuts) or manicures, and, if you want anything other than basic care (showers/meals/medication), you will likely need to pay for it privately. Spiritual and psychological support are practically nonexistent, and things like physiotherapy or speech therapy are rarely provided.

Because staffing ratios are poor in most residences, activities are limited. If an older adult is not particularly social, there won't be staff to adjust and provide 1:1 activities or support to fit that person's personality. Yes, an older adult will have something to do at some point, but if the person needs immediate help getting to the bathroom, or could benefit from playing an hour of Scrabble with someone, or want to lie down and need help getting into bed, there will likely be a wait time. This is why many people choose to pay a private nurse's aide or companion to spend several hours (a day) with an older adult to ensure an older person doesn't have to wait for what I consider assistance with a basic need.

> **Preparing for future housing is essential when we *Plan for Aging Well*. We must approach our eventual needs with a rational mind and make a financial plan to ensure we can get everything we need.**

If you want more information, visit www.stephanieerickson.ca. You can download the *Relocation Toolkit* to help you understand how to evaluate which type of residence is best for your loved one and how to monitor care on an ongoing basis.

Home Care

I think I've made my point that most people want to stay at home whenever possible. So how can we do that safely when we have health, mobility, and possibly cognitive problems? Home care.

There are many advantages to having someone come into your home and support you. First off, you're in your home! You have your bed. Your things. Your routine. Plus, you have constant interaction and attention focused on your needs, likes, and dislikes. You don't have to eat a shepherd's pie for dinner on Wednesday night if you don't want to (I see this on a lot of menus at residences). This may sound good to you, shepherd's pie. But after the 10th Wednesday in a row of eating the same thing, it may not have the same appeal. And what if you're a vegetarian? Or you have celiac disease? Then what?

Help at home can be for domestic tasks such as cleaning and food preparation, but it can also be more personal such as assistance with showering, dressing, medication administration, walking assistance, etc. Home care can also be about companionship and cognitive stimulation.

As you can imagine, this kind of help is not inexpensive. Hourly rates can run between $20 and $30 an hour depending on whether the assistance is for one person or two, and if it is strictly companionship or if it's for personal care, which requires someone with more training. If a person requires a licensed nurse for a particular procedure or health problem, the price goes up considerably. Prices vary based on location as well. Most companies require a minimum number of hours. In the end, it's on average at least $40,000 a year for 40 hours a week. But what if someone needs overnight care as well? This is why so many individuals end up moving. It is very expensive to stay home. If you are looking for resources or ways to find and bring care into your home, visit www.stephanieerickson.ca and you can download my *Home Care Toolkit*, which has strategies and a step-by-step guide.

If you find a live-in caregiver, that is sometimes more affordable. But, you have to consider that this person requires a room and bathroom as well as a few days off each week, so the family will have to make other arrangements on those days. It can be done but it isn't easy. In addition, this person will be considered an "employee" so you will need to consider what implications that has for the way in which you issue salary, benefits, vacation time, and of course, taxes. Make sure you check with your accountant and lawyer before you move someone into your house to minimize any potential risks.

If you choose to have in-home help there are risks. What if this person is abusive? Or steals? Or just doesn't show up and leaves your mom stranded? Can you trust a complete stranger to take care of your aging relative? Will you be able to concentrate at work knowing someone whom you barely know is with your mom? Would you feel the same level of (mis)trust if your parent was in a residence?

Using a home care agency comes with some checks and balances since at least this person (you hope) was vetted and trained and is supervised, and if there is a problem there is some accountability. I know many families, however, who have hired someone privately, and for cash, based on a personal referral and have had great success.

When bringing someone into the home it may take a few attempts before you find someone who is a good match with your relative's personality and skills. If your dad is a quiet man and you bring in a chatterbox, it may drive him crazy. But it also may perk him up and he could find it entertaining. You never know how personalities connect, and you may need to go through a few tries before you hit gold.

It may also be necessary to be very specific about what you expect from this person. Some caregivers take initiative and are very creative. Others will spend hours staring at the television alongside your parents and literally do nothing unless asked specifically. Don't be afraid to speak up and make a list of what you expect. Surprise drop-in visits are not a bad idea either.

This service can also be brought into a private or public residence. As I said earlier, I have seen far too many seniors slumped over in wheelchairs doing absolutely nothing for hours on end. I have heard many complaints from families about the wait time to have a protective undergarment changed, or their parent's discomfort in having to take a shower in the afternoon because of "scheduling" when their entire life they took one first thing in the morning.

For these reasons and more, families often hire private help in a residence or hospital to ensure that their parents have cognitive stimulation and personal attention when they need it. When my father-in-law (not the one with dementia) was having cancer treatments in the hospital, my husband and I paid for private care to be there because I knew that when he needed something, he needed it immediately. I did not want to make him wait or stress his wife out having to run around looking for staff and fighting for basic care.

You can also bring other types of support into the home as well. As a social worker, I make home visits all the time. I know physiotherapists and occupational therapists and nurses who do the same, all on a fee for service basis. There are doctors who can do this, but they are harder to find. In terms of spiritual support, you can ask a local church, synagogue, or mosque (or other religious institution) if they offer home visits. If they don't, there are some chaplains who make home visits for a fee, if you can find them.

The home environment is a great place to be when we are getting older. If you can be there safely with all of the support you need, it is a great option.

> **The bottom line is whether you move or stay home, if you need help, there are likely not enough community or government resources to meet your needs. You will have to pay.**

If you want more information visit www.stephanieerickson.ca, and you can download the *Home Care Toolkit* to help you understand how to find, hire, and supervise private care in your home.

I have to pay for this too? The Incidentals

One thing that we often forget to plan for is all of the "and this is not covered either" costs. If an older adult needs a cane or walker or wheelchair, does the government cover it? Does insurance? Or is it out of pocket?

Most of the items below are out-of-pocket expenses that are not covered by health insurance:

- Mobility devices (cane, walker, wheelchair)
- Equipment in the home (grab bars, raised toilet seat, special lounge chair, hospital bed, etc.)
- Safety systems (home alarms, personal alarms, sensors)
- Medication, vitamins
- Personal items (protective undergarments, which are also known as adult diapers)
- Special diets (diabetes, gluten-free, etc.)
- Medical supplies (needles, bandages, oxygen, etc.)
- Transportation (taxis, parking for medical appointments and hospitalizations, gas, hiring a companion for appointments)
- Travel (plane/airfare/gas/hotel) for adult children who come into town to assist their parent
- Professional fees (legal, psychological, social services, physiotherapy, etc.)
- Moving fees

When we are looking at the cost of growing older, some of these things on the list may not apply to your family. But what if they do? If you need to drive your parent to the hospital three times a week for dialysis, are you supposed to pay $20 for parking each time or should your parent pay? How will you have this conversation?

All of these things should be considered when we think about and *Plan for Aging Well*. I understand we cannot predict how many extras our family members will need. But making sure that some funds are set aside for just these types of unpredictable expenses can save a lot of headaches.

Sign on the Dotted Line

Jennifer phoned me in a panic. Her father, who had been having headaches for the past six months, refused to go to the doctor. After a fainting incident he admitted himself to the hospital and was soon diagnosed with Stage 4 brain cancer. Within a week he could no longer communicate clearly, and his family and the doctors couldn't confirm if he could understand what they were saying.

He didn't have a Living Will. He didn't have a Last Will and Testament.

Since he was divorced, his kids had to decide how to proceed. Should they authorize surgery to see if the tumor could be removed? Should they authorize radiation to see if the tumor would shrink so that they can at least have some more time with him? Or did their dad prefer palliative care? To make matters worse, one of the three children wanted to try everything, while the other two thought palliative care was the way to go. Who was in charge, and who got to decide?

> **Please, please, please make sure that you and your parents have a Living Will and Last Will and Testament in place.**

As a social worker, this situation is one that I hear about daily. It is also one that I experienced. You see, despite my work and my full understanding of what should be done, I couldn't convince my father of it. I had tried repeatedly to speak to him about legal documents and getting his affairs in order, but he refused to discuss it. I was relentless in my pursuit, but I couldn't force him to do anything.

On December 27, 2011, he died of a massive heart attack. He didn't have a Last Will and Testament and he never discussed funeral arrangements with my sister and me. We made the decision to have him cremated and to have a rock and roll party in his honor. I'm not sure what his sisters thought of our plan, but my sister and I feel that we did right by our dad. He also didn't really have any money, so splitting almost nothing 50/50 wasn't complicated.

Fortunately, my sister and I are very close and we were able to make joint decisions without ruining our relationship. But this isn't always the case.

When important legal documents are not prepared, families are left stranded without even the smallest unreliable compass to lead them out. Trust can be destroyed and relationships mutilated, and guilt and confusion may linger for years to come.

I know. It's not pleasant to think about getting old or dying or leaving your family behind. But it is a fact of life. You are a few minutes older than you were when you picked up this book. You can't escape these realities no matter how hard you try.

One of the most important and loving acts we can do for our families is to put our wishes in writing. Why do I include this information in the Aging Pocketbook chapter? Because not having our wishes in writing has a direct impact on our financial well-being. We need to make sure that the money we have earned in our lifetime is protected and managed appropriately. We must ensure that there are funds designated to meet our future needs. Just read this chapter again if you need convincing as to how much aging can cost.

These documents have different names in different countries. But these are the documents you need:

- A document authorizing someone to manage your property and assets (commonly called a Power of Attorney)
- A document authorizing someone to make healthcare decisions on your behalf (commonly called an Advanced Directive, Healthcare Surrogate, Durable Power of Attorney for Healthcare, or Medical Power of Attorney)
- A document outlining your expectations of the type of care you wish to receive (commonly called a Living Will or Healthcare Directive). It should include:
  - Housing options
  - Home care options
  - Treatment options (feeding tube, DNR orders, etc.)
  - Funeral instructions
- A document regarding the dispersing of your assets after your death (commonly called a Last Will and Testament or Trust)
- Refer to the Resources at the end of the book for links to forms available in the U.S. and Canada

Having these documents is helpful, but it's only the beginning. You cannot predict every situation, and there are many crises that can occur that leave families confused about how to respond. When families aren't quite sure which decision to make, they're likely to end up arguing with everyone, trying to insist his or her opinion is the one that matters. For example, just because a document says "DNR" does not necessarily translate into every situation. If I'm in a car accident, do I want a DNR order? Or do I want the DNR order to apply if I have a terminal illness?

> **This is why it's crucial for families to discuss these issues in advance to ensure that the legal documents we put into place are understood fully and leave little room for interpretation.**

In addition, I highly recommend that your legal documents are as specific as possible and include details that will help your family work together as cooperatively as possible. You will want your family to know your feelings about tube feeding, and DNR, and terminal illness. You will want them to understand your priorities of living environments should you fall ill. If an older adult can no longer consent or participate in discussions and make decisions, whoever is his or her representative should do the following, and these points should be put into writing.

In my experience, these extra clauses can be very helpful and reduce family conflict:

- Transparency to all beneficiaries regarding the use of funds for care
- Funds allotted for family who take time off work to provide care and support
- Funds allotted for family who must travel to assist with caregiving responsibilities
- Requirements for regular updates by the primary caregiver regarding the aging relative's functioning (email, phone calls, texts)
- If applicable, some decisions require the input of others, perhaps by majority decision
- An intermediary person named to facilitate communication if some family members are in conflict. Funds set aside for a professional mediator if conflict arises and no agreement can be reached

> **This illustrates the concept of *Plan for Aging Well*. We must *create* what we want through open communication, clear documents, and transparency.**

Sick Days

When a relative is getting older and he or she needs support, who is going to provide it? Well, if you haven't guessed it by now, I'd be surprised. It's the family.

Most of the adult children with whom I work have full-time jobs. They call me from work, spending 45 minutes explaining their situation and asking for support. They take off a few hours, a half day or a full day, to meet with me and their parent. Many take a leave of absence because trying to manage their work responsibilities with the time commitment and emotional stress of helping a family member is too much. And so many use their own money to pay for care their parents cannot afford.

What happens when you miss work? Do you lose your job? If you use your sick days on behalf of someone else, what happens when you get sick? If you take a leave, are you still covered by insurance? How do you pay your expenses? During your time off, are you still accumulating savings for your retirement? If you use your own money to pay for the care of a family member, who will pay for you if you need help down the road?

Aging is not an individual process. It is a family experience, and all members of the family will be financially impacted.

So many adult children tell me about the amount of money they have sacrificed to help their parents. "She did so much for me. It's the least I can do" is not an uncommon statement. I respect that and understand it. We don't want to turn our backs on our parents.

However, it is essential to recognize that we also need to prepare for our own aging and plan ahead so that we too can have all the support and care available when we need it. Please don't ignore the reality that your financial support for a loved one has a direct impact on your own care in the future.

For many adult children, money is already flying out the door to pay for sending their children to university, or to help pay for their daughter's wedding, or perhaps to support a child who has a mental or physical illness and cannot work. We all have current financial obligations that cannot be ignored.

> **It is important that you consider your needs too, and have an open and honest discussion with your aging relatives to ensure that they have communicated their wishes and expectations to you, and that you are honest with them about your own needs and financial limitations.**

CHAPTER 7

Team Caregiver

When we think of a caregiver we usually envision either a family member or a professional, such as a nurse's aide. Both are accurate. A caregiver, by definition, is someone who provides support to another person. Many people define caregiving as providing personal care assistance by helping someone get dressed or take a shower. These are some of the tasks that caregivers undertake, it's true. But caregiving is so much more than this description.

Most family caregivers describe how their role as a caregiver crept up on them in such subtle ways they never noticed. It seemed that one day they were living their own independent life and then, suddenly, they were going to their parents' house daily to make sure they were eating dinner and to give them their medication.

The role of caregiver often starts in small increments, so we may not consider what we are doing as caregiving. Your parents want you to attend a meeting with their financial advisor. That's not caregiving? Your mom has a doctor's appointment and she cannot drive afterwards because she needs a minor procedure. Of course, you agree to take her. That's not caregiving either? This is just what we do for our parents? These are the first small indications that your parents are aging and they are beginning to need your help. These actions *are* caregiving. They may be intermittent and simple, but they still count.

Caregivers, in my experience, are individuals who help someone even in small and infrequent ways. I think it is important that we acknowledge what we are doing and label it. Yes, I said it. Labels can be helpful in some situations. Our society seems so afraid of labeling people that we have swung to the other pendulum and avoid identifying with a particular group. But sometimes labels are good when they help us realize we're not alone in dealing with these challenges.

> Acknowledging our role as a caregiver can help us manage stressors that come with the role. We are more likely to seek help when we have named the problem and can be more direct in finding a solution. It also gives us a vocabulary to connect with others who have a shared experience, to define our needs more clearly and to seek help.

I've often heard the argument that some family members don't want to consider themselves caregivers because they are doing it out of love, and calling it "caregiving" somehow trivializes it or makes it too impersonal. Acknowledging that you have a formal role in someone's life is not impersonal. I believe it is just the opposite. It is a verbal statement of commitment. You care about someone and are involved in his life in order for him to live as autonomously and safely as possible. It's a beautiful thing and far from impersonal.

If this applies to you, say this out loud. "**I am a caregiver.**"

Again. "**I am a caregiver.**"

Now take a breath and read on.

It Takes a Village—Twice

We have all heard the saying that "it takes a village to raise a child." Well, the same applies to supporting an aging person. One person cannot be solely responsible for satisfying all of the aging person's needs.

One person can never meet the needs of another on her own. When we are aging, there are many physical, emotional, spiritual, and psychological changes that transform us, sometimes slowly and sometimes quickly. Family caregivers have to be on their toes to manage rapid changes and acute health crises. With each change, each problem, each setback, a caregiver must reach out to healthcare professionals for advice and guidance, and to other family members or friends for support. At least, this is how it should be.

Many family caregivers feel isolated as if they alone must bear the burden of caring for their loved one. It is sad and disheartening that our society and healthcare systems are so disconnected and broken that we are not working as a well-oiled machine. It's not like aging and the challenges of aging are new. I mean, really. We've been aging for millennia. You would think we would have a better handle on it.

Touchdown!

I have always loved football. It started back when I was a young girl and watched my father pace the room engrossed in the Rams' games, commenting on plays and shouting out at the refs. He knew every player and every statistic. But, it wasn't until my son started playing the game that a deep admiration and appreciation for the sport took hold. I learned so much about teamwork and all of the hard work and preparation it takes to inspire and motivate a team to victory.

One of the ways to approach caregiving is the same way you would if you were putting together a football team. First, the team must have a head coach. The head coach knows what outcomes are desired and will work to lead the team in this direction. A win in football is easy to determine and is based purely on a score. Obviously, there is no score in caregiving, but wins can be clearly defined by the care recipient, and the team can be motivated to earn that win. The head coach sees the big picture and long-term plan, and can recruit and lead star players and assistant coaches he trusts to make up the offense, defense, and special teams.

The head coach on a caregiving team is the person who needs care (also known as the client, care recipient, resident, etc.). The care recipient is the person most invested in the outcomes, lives with the problems 24/7, and knows the most about what he or she wants. The care recipient never misses a game. She or he attends all of the appointments, is intimately involved in every play, and suffers the losses more than anyone. But no head coach can lead a team to victory alone, especially one who is limited due to physical, cognitive, or psychological challenges. There are too many moving parts, and a smart head coach finds other key leaders and team members to ensure victory.

Every team needs an offense, a group of players who are focused on moving forward to achieve victory. The offensive coordinator must be thinking two steps ahead and knows how to call the plays with a keen insight and proactive approach in consideration of all of the blockades and barriers that could emerge. This is the primary caregiver, the person who provides the majority of care or spends the most amount of time with the care recipient. The primary caregiver sees it all—the good, the bad, and the ugly— and can give you the reality of the situation at any moment. The head coach has to trust the offensive coordinator to call the plays, knowing that it takes a variety of attempts and paths to get to the end zone.

A strong defensive team stays on their toes, ready to step in when needed. The defensive coordinator is someone who, under pressure, can respond with precision to attack each problem without hesitation. This person has the unique vision to see the set-up of an offensive play and adjust quickly. This is usually the primary physician who understands what is realistic and what medical treatments are available, and has the research and playbook to react and support the plan.

Each team must also have a special teams coach. This person is a problem solver ready to respond to a last-minute complication with a tailor-made intervention that can be executed smoothly and quickly. When the offensive plan doesn't work, this person is ready to jump in with an alternative. If a punt is delivered, this person is ready to catch and run for the end zone to make the play happen. In terms of caregiving, the special teams coach member may be a social worker, care manager, nurse, healthcare advocate, or, of course, a family member.

Each of these coaches is responsible for recruiting other key players, holding them accountable, and encouraging them to execute the plan flawlessly. Those key players are other family members and friends as well as other healthcare professionals. These roles are not cemented in stone. Be flexible. "Hire" your coaches for their skills and put them in the role that fits their skill set as well as their personality. You may envision them in one position, but if it's not a match to their skill set, interest, or comfort level, they will not be able to perform optimally.

If you watch a professional football game you will see how a skilled team works as a well-oiled machine. A play is called for every down, and there is always an offensive plan. The head coach communicates with his coaches, who in turn communicate with his quarterback, who then communicates the plan to the team, who lines up ready to execute at the quarterback's call. Everyone has their role and knows where to go.

The leader of the team is the quarterback. This is the person who understands the big picture and can inspire the team to victory. The quarterback must be able to think quickly on his feet so if a long pass was called but the receiver is covered, he can adjust and throw a quick short pass to someone else who is ready and waiting. The quarterback must remain calm and, no matter what happens, shake off the last play and get ready for the next one. Often, the quarterback is a social worker or care manager.

The best teams aren't the ones that have only one star player. Sure, that helps if you have someone who can seemingly do it all. But what if that player gets hurt? Where will the team be now if there is only one player who can lead them to victory? Each caregiving team must have several players who are competent, efficient, invested, and committed to the goal to make it work.

After all, if you have the No. 1 running back in the league and the offensive line doesn't block and open a hole, the running back will never gain yards. When the quarterback throws a bomb downfield, he must have confidence that he can launch the pass ahead of the receiver knowing that he won't break stride and he will be there to catch the pass. Caregiving also requires having a plan, executing it, and trusting your team to be there when you need them.

Each of the coaches and team players should be chosen by the care recipient. She is the head coach who decides who she wants to be in her organization. She can add or release anyone as she sees fit, and all individuals within the organization should respect her plan and goals.

It is quite spectacular to watch a professional football team work in unison, everyone executing their role with one plan and one common goal. This should be how caregiving works.

Team Discussions

From my football analogy above, you get the point. There are many team players and we must try to act in unison. Many caregivers fall into a trap thinking that they should be driving the care and choices. Don't get me wrong. If a person has moderate or severe dementia, she may not be able to understand and appreciate her situation and make decisions. However, even someone with dementia can make some choices, no matter how small, and take a role in her care. Certainly, the care recipient, well in advance of having care needs, could have communicated her wishes in writing and discussed them with her family so the goal is clear, even if the care recipient can no longer actively participate in its execution.

Let's focus on the conversations that should be happening about planning to meet the care recipient's needs. Since the care recipient should lead the way, it is extremely important that he has communicated his wishes, expectations, fears, opinions, and choices in advance, in writing and on an ongoing basis if he is able to express himself. We all have the right to determine what kind of care we want, which intervention we prefer, where we want to live, and who we want to help us. Believe me, if these conversations are not had in advance, or if they are held privately and not as a team, messages get crossed, anger erupts, and not only the care recipient suffers. The entire family will suffer.

Refer back to Chapter Six, The Aging Pocketbook. I discussed many of the essential documents needed to preserve family harmony and to ensure that a person's wishes are understood and respected. Without these wishes clearly indicated in writing and in conversations with all family members, there is bound to be misinterpretations and guesswork and the person may not have his or her needs met in the way the person would have wanted. I have seen many, many families thrown into conflict by vague or nonexistent directives.

These discussions are painfully hard to initiate for most families. On one side of my family, my dad would never discuss aging, no matter how many times I tried to initiate a conversation. He never told my sister or me how he wanted us to support him if he fell ill. Any time I brought it up, he started to sweat, reminding me of the days when he taught me how to drive a stick shift. He refused to participate in any conversation related to aging, illness, or finances. Thankfully, at least he said to my sister and me countless times that he trusted us and that we always make good decisions. It wasn't nearly enough, but it was something.

My grandma, on the other hand, is an open book. She invited each family member to tour her home and write our names on stickers to place under items to ensure we are gifted with things that are meaningful to us after she dies. She has a lawyer with whom she meets regularly, and all of her legal documents are in place. She has gone over her wishes with her kids—and even changed them later in life (preferring cremation over burial).

My grandma proactively chose her autonomous seniors residence for several reasons. A key reason was that it is directly connected to a long-term care facility should she need it. She has thought it all out, prepared in advance, and shared her plan. She voices her opinion on all matters and expects, rightfully so, that her children support her in achieving her goals. At ninety-seven, despite her petite body and quiet voice, she is a force who knows what she wants and shares her opinion without qualms.

My mom is somewhere in the middle. I know who her attorney is but I've never met with him. We have briefly discussed her funeral plans (although I don't know the details, only that they are somewhere in her papers) and I have a broad understanding that I am the executor of her Last Will and Testament. But that's all I know. She remarried when I was in my 20s. She has not been fully transparent with what she wants and expects, and truthfully, I'm not sure she knows herself. But if she hasn't been clear with me, has she been clear with my stepdad? If not, we could have some conflict down the line if we disagree on care, housing, burial options, or whatever. I am in a continual conversation with her and encourage her to think about her future and express her expectations clearly and concisely.

One of my clients said to me recently, "My dad was clear he didn't want me to tell my brothers that he named me as his Power of Attorney. He wanted his privacy. But now that he can no longer communicate, my brothers think I haven't been transparent and they are angry and resentful."

> **Being vague or reluctant to share details about what you expect should you need help is a recipe for disaster.**

One thing that I often see in my clinical practice is a lack of transparency with family members. Many care recipients have outlined their wishes in writing and may have even had discussions with a family member, but not all family members. When it comes to siblings of an aging parent, I have been a witness to horrific conflicts, lost funds to attorneys, legal battles, and shattered relationships as a result of one-sided, secret conversations.

In my clinical work, I conduct psychosocial evaluations to determine if a person retains the mental capacity to make decisions for himself. Most of my clients have dementia. As part of this process, I read legal documents, such as a Power of Attorney, constantly. Time and time again when I reach out to my client's adult children, I hear stories of betrayal and secrecy. For example, one adult child may allege that his sibling brought their mother to an attorney to draft a legal document in secret and with the intention of exclusion. When scenarios like this occur, whether or not they are even true, these adult children who need to be aligned to make joint decisions fracture their relationship. Who suffers? The older adult.

> **In order to be a team and approach caregiving as a unified, well-oiled machine, we must share our expectations with every team player, even if some will be angry or resentful. If you wait, it will absolutely be worse in times of crisis.**

None of us like to be lied to. Wouldn't you prefer, even if the truth hurts, to be respected enough to hear it? I know I would. At the very root of team caregiving is the concept that all team members, no matter how involved or uninvolved they are, must be informed by the care recipient of what is to come down the line. This is the care recipient's job. Do your job and put your wishes, expectations, and instructions in writing and have those necessary conversations.

When care recipients outline their expectations and clearly explain them to their family, the family can advocate on their behalf and make sure that their plan is implemented. There are so many moving parts in caregiving, and without clear communication and instructions, things can get twisted. You can find a guide on questions to initiate conversation in the Caregiving Toolkit at www.stephanieerickson.ca

Who is on the team?

A caregiving team is comprised of every person who is involved in care, no matter the size of their role.

The caregiving team consists of the care recipient, primary caregiver, doctors, nurses, nurse's aides, social worker, physiotherapist, occupational therapist, speech therapist, pharmacist, dietitian, advocate, care manager, and any other healthcare professional. It can also include family members, friends, neighbors, or volunteers. Caregivers do not need to live locally. If the primary caregiver is a spouse, and the children of the care recipient live out of town but come into town occasionally to help, or speak to the care recipient's spouse regularly to provide emotional support, they too are caregivers.

The solid base of any caregiving team must include consent to disclose information. Anyone other than the care recipient is not allowed to receive information without the written authorization of the care recipient, which is done in a variety of ways depending on the state or province in which you live.

In some locations, you may need to sign a specific form that the provider has generated. For example, some doctors have their own form that they expect family to sign and will not except a standardized form printed online. Some hospitals require people to go to the medical archive department (where they store all of the medical records and documents within a hospital or other healthcare setting) to sign a release. Other healthcare professionals will accept an online-generated form. Make sure to ask the provider what he or she will accept at the onset of your contact with him or her.

This must be a priority for care recipients to trust their caregivers and allow for the sharing of information. It makes it much easier for everyone to communicate and develop and implement a feasible plan.

The Care Recipient

As discussed in the football analogy, the care recipient is the head coach. She is the person who decides what she would like in terms of interventions, care, support, treatment, financial expenditures, etc. I frequently attend care plan meetings with healthcare professionals and caregivers. The care plan is the formalized outline of what will be offered and how it will be offered.

For example, a care plan may include goals related to mobility, such as "Increase the patient's ability to maintain balance and walk unassisted for three feet." The intervention offered may be physiotherapy twice a week and perhaps a recommendation of adding handrails in the home. Care plans can address everything from nutrition to mobility to increased support systems to skin integrity, and a specific professional would be implemented in the care planning, such as a physiotherapist in the example above.

Unfortunately, too often, the healthcare providers and the caregiver talk about the plan in front of the care recipient but don't include him in the process. If I were the care recipient, I would probably shout out, "Hello? Does anyone see I'm sitting here listening? Don't I have a voice?" We all must remember that the care recipient has a right to decide on his care plan. Without his input, nothing should be created or implemented. An obvious exception is when the care recipient can no longer communicate his needs and his healthcare surrogate (legal representative) is advocating on his behalf.

The Primary Family Caregiver

In most situations, one family member or close friend has taken on the role of primary caregiver. The primary caregiver is the person who is most involved in the day-to-day care and understands all of the details of the care recipient's situation. If the care recipient is married, it's usually the spouse.

Some families choose to have adult children step in and take on this main role, especially when it comes to communicating with healthcare professionals. Adult children are typically more knowledgeable about technology (emails, video conferencing, printing/scanning documents, online payments, etc.) and this can help in speeding up communications or making things more efficient. Still, if there is a spouse, she or he should be running the show and delegating to the adult children, assuming this is what the care recipient wants.

Additional Caregivers

Caregivers can be anyone. If a person has many children, all of them would be considered caregivers. If there is a niece or nephew involved, she or he are caregivers. There are also paid caregivers, such as home care assistants, who are able to offer information and insight into particular situations. Perhaps there are neighbors or family friends around helping to bring meals or drive to medical appointments. Anyone who has stepped up and offers consistent help can be considered a caregiver.

The Doctor

Aside from the care recipient and caregiver, many healthcare professionals come in and out of the care recipient's life. Depending on the role of the healthcare professional, care recipients and caregivers may feel intimidated and reluctant to speak up.

For many people, an M.D. has all the answers and should not be questioned. I am not minimizing the extensive training and experience physicians have. But do not forget that they are human. They make mistakes. They have experience but not *your* exact experience, and it is important that you share your perception and experience with each doctor you meet.

I have heard many stories and I have witnessed this myself how many people are unwilling to question a doctor or ask for more information, or to refute what she is saying, or admit they do not quite understand what is being said, especially older generations who see a medical doctor as the all-knowing Oz who is never to be questioned or doubted. I tell caregivers and care recipients all the time not to forget that this is their life, not the doctor's, and they should understand and agree with every plan that is put into place.

> A care recipient and caregiver should be heard by their doctor and they are integral to the care planning process. Only the care recipient and/or caregiver know what is realistic and what is not. Do not be afraid to speak up.

Many people have multiple doctors with different specialties, which can make care planning all the more challenging. Who is in charge of the overall health and medical plan? Which disease is taking priority? Which medications are more important than others? Depending on the "system" in which you are seeking care, medical records may not be electronic or accessible by other professionals, which is not ideal.

This makes it even more essential for the caregiver and/or care recipient to be the head coach who ensures that all of the other coaches and players are communicating with one another. Make sure you ask for written summaries, or take notes yourself and share these documents with the team so that there are no wires crossed or interventions that are put into place that will derail the overall goals.

Pharmacist

Often pharmacists are not considered as part of the caregiving team. They should be. Not only are they clearly experts on medication and side effects, but if one pharmacist is included on the team (this means not getting different medications from different locations), she can ensure that there are no adverse interactions between medications prescribed by different physicians unknowingly. Also, you must inform the pharmacist of every over-the-counter drug, vitamin, or "natural" product that is being taken as there can be adverse effects that could be preventable. In addition, pharmacists can provide insight into medication compliance (particularly related to those with cognitive problems), which can be very helpful for families to ensure safety.

Nurse

I love nurses. Not only do they understand the disease and its impact on the patient, they are emotionally connected with the care recipient and family and a direct link to the doctor. Most nurses spend time with their care recipients to get to know him or her. They truly understand a care recipient's experience, and they also understand the role caregivers play in keeping the care recipient healthy and supported. Doctors look to their nurses to provide a quick summary of pressing concerns and will often respond to their nurses much quicker than if a care recipient contacts them directly. Make sure to ask the nurse for emergency procedures and the fastest way to get a hold of the doctor.

In this section, nurse refers to a registered nurse (RN) or a nurse practitioner, licensed practical nurse (LPN), or registered nursing assistant (RNA).

Orderlies

The true front-line workers are orderlies. They are the person who is generally with a care recipient for more hours a day or week than any other healthcare professional. They provide real hands-on assistance such as helping someone bathe or get dressed, get fed, or change a protective undergarment, or help a person move from one location to another.

Often orderlies are left out of discussions and care planning. They don't hold the same credibility or authority as other healthcare professionals, likely because they don't have a degree or license. But in my opinion, orderlies can provide a wealth of information and are the backbone of any treatment plan. They should be respected and included.

In this section an orderly can also be referred to as a nurse's aide, attendant, personal support worker, or, for all intents and purposes, a companion.

Social Worker

Full disclosure. I'm biased about the value of social workers because I am one! I am aware of how much we know and are capable of doing, from understanding dementia and other diseases, the impact on the care recipient's functioning, the implications for the primary caregiver, the toll it takes on the entire family system, and the role each healthcare professional plays. In interdisciplinary meetings we are often the calming voice mediating the discussion to ensure the care recipient's needs are met because our client is the care recipient, and we do whatever we can to understand what our client wants. We advocate in and out of healthcare systems to ensure goals are realistic and achievable and that they are met. Social workers, in my opinion, have the best pulse on the overall situation and can communicate it to other professionals and between family members.

Physical Therapist/Physiotherapist

If the care recipient had surgery or an injury, or just needs to build up strength, mobility, and flexibility, a physical therapist or physiotherapist (PT) will be part of the team. Generally, a PT is a short-term team member. She will evaluate a person's physical strength and create a plan to follow to rebuild that strength, get the care recipient walking again, or whatever the goal is. Typically, a PT would evaluate a diagnosis (i.e., left hip fracture) to make sure that the plan fits the problem. A PT doesn't read x-rays or scans, but a summary of these findings can be helpful.

It is important for a PT to know the medications someone is taking; some drugs can cause balance problems or other risks, so the plan may need to be adjusted. For the most part, PTs do not get involved directly with the family, other than scheduling and some instruction on teaching exercises that can be continued at home. Equipment may be recommended by a PT as well for the care recipient and/or the home environment.

Occupational Therapist

An occupational therapist (OT) is skilled at understanding a person's physical, functional, and cognitive capabilities in his own environment. She will test the care recipient with hands-on activities, such as cooking an egg or filling out a check to really understand what the care recipient can and cannot do. OTs make recommendations on how to outfit a home to ensure the person's safety. With these evaluations, it is necessary for the OT to communicate with the primary caregiver to make sure the recommendations are clear, easy to follow, and realistic considering the care recipient's specific home environment. Often OTs are involved in different stages in a person's life, especially if the care recipient has a progressive disease that changes his overall functioning over time.

Dietitian

So many people underestimate how much a dietary consult can change things for a care recipient, especially from a dietitian who specializes in older adults. Our body needs fuel and the right kind of fuel to help us maximize our energy, and health is essential. As we age, we lack certain minerals and vitamins to help us function as we had in our younger years. A dietary plan can do wonders for a person's overall health and functioning. A skilled dietitian will consider budget and ability to shop and cook, as well as understand health implications and risks of any nutritional changes. If a care recipient requires a modified diet due to difficulty swallowing or other issues such as celiac disease, diabetes, or lactose intolerance, a dietician will be instrumental in putting together a solid nutritional plan.

Speech and Language Pathologist

For many older adults, speech and language can be affected after a stroke. In addition, some strokes or other illnesses can lead to dysphagia (difficulty swallowing). A speech and language pathologist or speech therapist will facilitate a swallow exam to determine if there is dysphagia and will make recommendations to the family, often in collaboration with a dietitian, about what foods to avoid and how to specially prepare diets of soft foods, pureed foods, and thickened liquids. A speech and language pathologist can also assist a person in gaining speech back, for example, after a stroke.

Recreational Therapist

A recreational therapist brings joy into the care recipient's life by creating opportunities for physical exercise, group and social activities, and cognitive stimulation. In a residence, this person is often referred to as the activities coordinator. (Note: an RT has a university degree, but often residence coordinators do not have this extensive training). A skilled recreational therapist will get to know a person's likes and dislikes as well as interests, strengths, and weaknesses. The RT will build an individualized plan for families to implement at home to provide stimulation. In a group environment, like a residence, the RT puts together an activity plan to meet the needs of the majority of residents. It will include exercise, games, discussions, and more.

Spiritual Advisor

Spirituality is the part of us that looks for meaning and brings us a sense of peace. Fulfilling this part of us is just as important as taking care of our physical health, and a spiritual advisor is one of the people who can understand and execute this plan. A spiritual advisor can be a chaplain, a priest, a rabbi, an imam, a minister, or any other person attached to a religious organization. A "spiritual coach" (or a version of this) is another form of support that many people find helpful.

A spiritual advisor should be a part of any care team. This person can ensure that important rituals such as observing the fast at Ramadan, lighting candles for Shabbat dinner, or taking communion are facilitated. For people who don't identify with a religion or its rituals, the spiritual advisor can still understand what brings meaning or peace to a person and put that plan into place. Discussions around a "higher power" can be initiated, as can other perspectives on how a person makes sense of the world. For example, if the ocean brings a person comfort, then the spiritual advisor can make sure there are sounds of waves played on a CD player and pictures of the ocean are hanging on the walls.

Geriatric Care Manager

In the U.S., there are certified geriatric care managers who have gone through training, and there is a certification process to obtain this designation. They must have the credentials and the practical experience to receive certification. Those who have gone through these programs have dedicated themselves to putting in the time through their formal education and practical experience to know their jobs well.

These individuals are typically social workers or nurses and can be a fantastic resource to help families navigate healthcare systems, facilitate family discussions, and find resources to help a care recipient and the caregivers.

Some of the certifications and certifying organizations include:

- Advanced Aging Life Professional from Aging Life Care Association (formerly known as the National Association of Geriatric Care Managers)
- Care Manager Certified from National Academy of Certified Care Managers
- Certified Case Manager from the Commission for Case Manager Certification
- Certified Advanced Social Work Case Manager or Certified Social Work Case Manager from the National Association of Social Workers
- Certified Geriatric Care Manager from the International Commission on Healthcare Certification

There are many other "designations" in the U.S. and Canada, but I caution families to be wary of certifications not on this list. While these individuals may have some knowledge and experience, many do not have any background related to nursing or social work. These certificates have been earned in hours vs. the years of training and practical experience earned with a degree.

I am *not* saying that they are not competent, but I do recommend working with someone who is certified based on education (minimum of a bachelor's degree in social work or nursing) who has completed internships or practicums with supervision and has extensive front-line experience. An educational degree also holds weight when these professionals work with other healthcare professionals. In addition, having a license with requirements for ongoing continuing education means a professional is likely to be kept up to date on new training and interventions. They also understand medical terminology and how interdisciplinary teams work. There is also an inherent accountability system that holds a professional accountable when they are licensed.

A care manager can be the quarterback to receive the play and then execute it smoothly. They help to navigate the system and make sure each wheel keeps spinning and moving forward, coordinating each step along the way. If you have the funds to hire a care manager to be the point person, I recommend you do so. This person can remain objective, which enables him to hear the information being presented by team members in a different way than a family member or care recipient does, since there is less emotional investment in the outcomes.

Advocate

An advocate, in its purest definition, is someone who represents another person's interest. In the healthcare world, advocates are individuals who speak up for vulnerable populations to the media, lawmakers, and healthcare systems demanding change and necessary support. Advocates can also work one-on-one with a care recipient or caregiver in the context of a complex healthcare system to ensure that the care recipient is receiving the care he wants and deserves and is available.

In the healthcare setting, many different individuals or family members can step into the role of advocate, but not in an official capacity. Some hospitals have their own patient advocate, but this often is the person who receives complaints. The ombudsman (discussed further below) can also be considered an advocate in residences and in some home care or other healthcare settings.

There is a growing profession of professional advocates emerging in the healthcare setting who are outside the "system" and not employed by the hospital or other healthcare setting. Many advocates have a background in nursing and social work and have the expertise through their education and experience to take on this role. Other advocates are those who have learned through their own personal experience how the system works or what a person may need.

As with my cautions related to geriatric care managers, I recommend that families work with an advocate who has a professional degree and experience behind them. GCMs with a license have credibility with other healthcare professionals, which can be very helpful. They also must follow strict ethical guidelines related to confidentiality and procedures, which improves the delivery of services and ensures appropriate actions. Advocates without a professional degree or license do not have continuing education requirements or a license that holds them accountable and ensures ethical guidelines are adhered to.

Relocation Specialist

Relocation specialists are a great resource. These professionals specialize in knowing the various private small and large residences within a community. A skilled relocation specialist will meet with healthcare providers, the patient, and the family to understand fully the patient's level of functioning and the type of short-term and long-term support needed. Based on this, the relocation specialist acts as a liaison for the family, showing them the residences most closely matched to the needs of the patient and within the patient's budget. This helps save the family endless hours of feeling overwhelmed and confused by all of the options available.

Organizations

It goes without saying that the organization or "system" that is providing care is also a vital team member. Any staff member who has information about your loved one or offers assistance to him or her should be included. Many of those staff members are listed above, but there may be additional team members that may not be there. Make sure to ask who is involved in caring for your aging relative at the hospital, rehabilitation facility, home care agency, residence, medical clinic, or community agency (for example, Meals on Wheels, an adapted transportation service, etc.).

If you would like more information about how to communicate with and document your interactions with healthcare professionals, visit www.stephanieerickson.ca. You can also download the toolkit Communication with Healthcare Professionals.

Lawyers

Lawyers can be very helpful in working with families and older adults. They are able to draft the various legal documents necessary to prepare and execute someone's wishes. I discussed these documents in detail in Chapter Six: The Aging Pocketbook. Lawyers can also step in to mediate family conflict and, if necessary, start legal proceedings to protect a senior from harm or abuse. Although some lawyers may have some experience in working in files related to a senior, there are a growing number of lawyers who specialize in elder law, and this area of law is an established concentration of practice. In the U.S., there is the National Academy of Elder Law Attorneys in which you can locate a lawyer in your area. The National Academy of Elder Law Attorneys' website lists those who are certified to practice elder law.

Lawyers cost money, and this is a barrier for many individuals who would like to seek their assistance. In the U.S., there are legal service programs funded under the Older Americans Act, and these referrals can be found by contacting a local area agency on aging, or by searching through *Eldercare Locator* online. In Canada, the Canadian Bar Association (CBA) has a "find an attorney" search engine that has a filter for "elder law" to find a specialist. In addition, on the CBA website there are links for Pro Bono and Legal Aid assistance.

Financial Advisors

At this point, I hope readers understand fully how important it is to plan in advance for our growing needs as we age. A financial advisor is an ally for you. A financial advisor can look at short- and long-term needs as an individual and as a couple. A skilled advisor will develop a realistic plan to ensure that you optimize your funds so that when you need them, they are available and sufficient. In addition, financial advisors have relationships with insurance advisors in order to consider if there are insurance products on the market that are right for your particular situation.

Houston, We Have a Problem

Things go wrong. It happens. Steps are missed in a procedure, communication lines are broken, or patients, in one way or another, are lost in a complex healthcare system. I always recommend that individuals and families speak up if they are dissatisfied with care or with a professional's actions. The first step is to go directly to the individual with whom you have an issue and start a dialogue. If it goes unresolved, seek this person's manager, or the head of the department in which they work. If those steps don't work, there are other options discussed below.

Ombudsman

The ombudsman is charged with the responsibility of representing the patient, the family, and the public. For example, in a hospital if a family is discouraged by the ongoing miscommunication among staff members that led to inappropriate or unsafe care delivery, the family can seek the help of the hospital ombudsman to look into the matter and resolve it.

Ombudsmen work in a variety of settings: hospitals, nursing homes, and other larger healthcare organizations. There are also ombudsmen associated with governmental branches but they typically do not step in for assistance; for example, in a hospital setting or long-term care home, since those organizations have their own internal ombudsman.

Long-term Care Ombudsman

In nursing homes, care is not always up to standards. There is abuse and neglect within residences that must be investigated so that organizations are held accountable. In every state in the U.S., there is a long-term care ombudsman that can be contacted for concerns related to care delivery or to report abuse or neglect. Call 1-800-252-2412, enter your zip code, and your county's local ombudsman contact information will be shared. In Canada, each province has its own long-term care ombudsman. You can find their phone number by simply searching "long-term care ombudsman" with the name of the province.

Patient Advocate Groups

In both the U.S. and Canada, there are patient advocate groups that can step in when you are having difficulty receiving proper care within the healthcare setting. As discussed in the Advocate section above, this person can help you understand the system and the complaint process, and help you communicate effectively your concerns. However, unlike the ombudsman, this person will not have the authority to step in and investigate complaints.

Conservatorship

There are times when an older adult is no longer able to represent himself on personal and/or financial matters due to a reduced cognitive capacity. In these situations, and when a legal document was not previously established, a family member can pursue legal steps to establish him or herself as a legal representative. Throughout the U.S. and Canada this role and the legal steps necessary to establish it will vary, as will the term used. The term may be "conservatorship," "substitute decision-maker," "legal guardian," "curator," or other term.

In most areas of North America, capacity to make decisions for oneself relates to one's property and financial matters, or to one's "person," which correlates to medical, personal, and housing decisions. A person may be capable in one aspect but not in another. In all regions, there is a court process that is initiated to establish in what way a person requires assistance and to determine who is the most appropriate person to take on that role. Check with an elder law attorney in your region to inform yourself on the steps required in your area.

Elder Abuse

Elder abuse. I've seen it. Many times. It's awful. Elder abuse can be physical, sexual, financial, neglect, exploitation, and psychological. It's under-reported by older adults because they are usually dependent on the abuser and fearful. It happens within families and with "friends" who appear on the scene to "help" a frail, elderly person. Even healthcare professionals can commit acts of abuse.

Most of the elder abuse calls I receive, unfortunately, are related to family members. For example, recently I received a call from a daughter of an older adult fearful about her mom's safety since her brother, who is a longtime drug addict, forced his way into their mom's home saying he would "take care" of her. In reality, he was having her sign checks in his name and leaving her alone all day as he walked the streets in search of drugs. Most of the families with whom I work really have the best interest of the senior at the forefront, but it's not always the case.

If you suspect any type of elder abuse, please report it. In the U.S., every state will have an Elder Protection Center, which you can contact and report your suspicions (or proof). You can call 1-800-677-1166 (Eldercare Locator) or the Administration for Community Living, which has a National Center on Elder Abuse. In Canada, each province has its own investigative body and process. You can locate this resource on the Government of Canada website. Of course, you can also contact the police directly and they can assist you.

Working 24/7

Caregiving is a full-time job in and of itself, Yet, many, many caregivers also have jobs. In the U.S., on average over half of caregivers work full-time. According to one study, 61 percent of caregivers were employed within the last year of their caregiving duties, and over half of these caregivers worked full-time (Caregiving in the U.S. Report, AARP, 2020). In Canada, 35 percent of the workforce provides informal, unpaid work as a caregiver while holding down a job. Approximately 1.6 million employees take time off and 10 percent give more than 30 hours of care a week (Report from the Employer Panel of Caregivers, 2015. "When Work and Caregiving Collide").

Employers and businesses do seem to be waking up to the working caregiving phenomenon, but they are definitely not anywhere near caught up. And for some caregivers who are not in "white-collar" businesses, there is absolutely no flexibility in working from home or making up hours on the weekend. When you work in a factory or in retail, your shift is your shift.

As discussed in Chapter Six: The Aging Pocketbook, it's not only seniors' pocketbooks that are impacted by an aging relative. As caregivers miss work their own financial and job security is impacted. Vacation and sick days are used for someone else's behalf. Promotions are missed. Colleagues are resentful. Retirement savings are reduced.

So, what do caregivers do? They half-work and half-provide care. Like many working parents, even without caregiving responsibilities, we feel like we are out of balance and no one gets the best of us. Not our work. Not our families. For caregivers, this feeling is even more profound as they add "loved one" or "parent" to the list of someone who is not getting the best of them.

You know who else is not getting the best of them? The caregivers. What I mean is that caregivers are so focused on doing what they can to attend to an aging relative, not lose their job, make sure their kids' needs are met, and keep their marriage afloat, they put themselves and their own health and well-being at the bottom of the priority list.

There is abundant evidence that working caregivers experience higher levels of stress and health problems as a result of balancing their caregiving and work responsibilities. They experience higher levels of mental health issues as well. Depression and anxiety are not uncommon among the family members who cross my path in my work.

As we know, there is a connection between mental health and physical health. Caregivers who are ill physically will miss work and use more insurance and disability benefits, leading to an increase in employers' costs. It makes business sense, in fact, for employers and businesses to develop creative plans to support caregivers.

In most healthcare environments, caregivers tend to be an overlooked group as healthcare professionals focus on the "patient." But if the patient's recovery or functioning directly depends on the contribution of caregivers, their physical and mental health needs must be addressed equally.

My hope is that the approach to supporting seniors shifts and caregivers' physical and mental well-being becomes an equal part of the equation. Healthcare professionals and systems must get creative in finding ways to meet the needs of both groups and intervene with support and resources for the entire family system.

CHAPTER **8**

Special Considerations

Our experiences directly shape the way in which we see the world regardless of our age. Each event, interaction, or experience that we have affects who we are in the next moment. On top of life's daily benign events, many of us have histories that include trauma and pain, and this magnifies how we see the world. Are we afraid? Have people hurt us? Betrayed us? Has our life been threatened? Are we alone?

As individuals get older, they become more dependent on others, which can make them feel vulnerable and scared. For those with a traumatic history and dementia, the world can become a very scary and lonely place.

Veterans

Veterans put their own well-being at risk in order to protect others. The experiences that many veterans have had are traumatic. Many witnessed horrific things, saw their comrades perish before their eyes, were asked to commit unspeakable acts in the name of freedom, and spent days, months, and years wondering if they would live to see another day. This history does not disappear from their core. Their bodies remember this pain and fear deep down. Even if their mind begins to fail, their bodies remember and react by any means necessary to protect themselves.

Sadly, veterans are one of society's neglected populations. Veterans are led to believe that they will be cared for and nurtured for the sacrifices that they made. Many are, I'm sure. But so many have post-traumatic stress disorder and other mental illnesses that are left untreated for years, and these individuals suffer needlessly. By the time these men and women reach old age, the trauma and fears of earlier years can have a direct impact on their overall functioning.

If veterans also have dementia, their memories can be mistaken as present-day circumstances, making life very scary and unmanageable. A veteran in pain can be thrown back to a foxhole where he was left for hours with a broken leg waiting for the medics to arrive. A screaming roommate can flood a veteran's mind with sounds of screaming comrades on the battlefield. An alarm bell in a residence can be reminiscent of the alarm sounding during an air raid. We must be sensitive to veterans and all they have sacrificed and experienced, and adjust our care and approach to show the compassion and respect they deserve.

Abuse Survivors

Whether a person experienced physical, sexual, or psychological abuse, those who have survived have overcome a unique set of circumstances that impacted their physical, emotional, and spiritual selves. As with all traumas, those who were abused have a multitude of ways in which they reacted during the abuse that shaped the way in which they view relationships, trust, and experiences. Some survivors developed PTSD, depression, or anxiety as a result of the abuse. Others seem to have moved past the memories, only to have them resurface in later years.

Imagine you were sexually abused by a neighbor as a young child. Now, someone you cannot recognize due to your dementia symptoms is trying to take your clothes off and guide you into the shower. Imagine you were beaten as a child and now someone is grabbing you, trying to move your body around into another position. Or, you were berated and told you were stupid as a child or as an adult, and now everyone is telling you that you don't know how to do something once again. It must be terrifying.

Some individuals may respond to the above triggers with physical and/or verbal aggression. Others may curl up in a ball and become passive and scared. We must be patient and understand that a survivor's body has memories that are sparked by no fault of his own, and the individual has been propelled into a fight or flight survival mode that helped him survive over the years.

Survivors of the Holocaust and Other Crimes Against Humanity

Have you ever boarded a train that was headed toward death? Have you ever been the only survivor in your family to have made it out alive from a situation that you all experienced simultaneously? Have you ever fled bombs sent into your village? Escaped famine and poverty that destroyed millions? Most likely, you haven't.

Individuals who have been witness to and experienced firsthand horrific crimes against humanity know deeper depths of pain than any human being can experience. To come out of those situations and go on to live a productive life shows a fighting spirit that I greatly admire and respect.

We must remember that these experiences and tragedies remain in people's minds forever. When a person has dementia and cannot process or understand the world around her, many things that seem non-threatening to most of us can be extremely frightening.

Imagine you survived the Holocaust by being sent away to live with a stranger and then were forced to stay inside that person's home. Now you are "sent away" to a residence and you cannot find an exit. Imagine a life of poverty and hunger, and now when you say you're hungry, you're told you just ate and you feel locked in a loop of looking for your next meal. Imagine you were separated from your family as a young child, reunited, and then once again, you are "looking" for them and they are nowhere to be found.

We must pay special attention to the uniqueness of survivors' experiences and show compassion and patience in how we address their needs. Those individuals who now have dementia find it hard to understand and communicate why they are reacting in a certain way. Something seemingly innocent to us feels like a punch in the chest to them, and we must be patient.

LGBTQ

Aging is hard in the best of circumstances. When you have been a part of a marginalized group your entire life, getting older can be even scarier. Imagine that through your life you were told you were different, unlovable, weird, or wrong. Now you are isolated in a nursing home with others who do not have a shared experience. There is a risk you will feel even more alone and vulnerable, or even worse, bullied or abused.

What if you have a partner of the same gender? Will he or she be welcome to visit you and show affection to you? Or will staff and other residents and families find your behavior "sick and disgusting"? If you are transgender and surgery scars are present, how will you feel if a staff member has to provide hygiene care? Will you be judged? What if you are physically a male but have always dressed as a woman? Will this be respected in your old age?

Currently, there are very few programs or residences that offer support tailored to the LGBTQ community. This community has done wonderful work in creating a feeling of togetherness and support, but they have often done so at a cost of being rejected by their families. Who will provide for them as they age if they have few family members and all of their peers are aging too?

It is important that professionals step up in these circumstances to ensure that individuals within this community are cared for and respected for who they are, and provide an environment and care in which they are supported and understood.

Visible Minorities

Have you ever been called a racial slur? Have you ever been denied service because of the color of your skin? Have you been discriminated against in accessing basic healthcare or other services? If you haven't, then you cannot begin to know the deep wounds that people of color have had to bear and survive.

Black and brown people, immigrants who may not speak English, and other visible minorities have been denied basic rights and justice that the majority of North Americans never question. People of color have been targeted and seen as "less than" not only throughout history, but in our current social, legal, financial, and political climate. This shapes the way in which they see the world because, in fact, their experiences are different from the majority of North Americans.

As a result, if a person's history is riddled with systemic racism, stereotyping, healthcare disparity, socioeconomic disparity, and discrimination, the way in which he or she, or his or her family members, seek and accept help will be impacted.

A member of a minority group may not ask for help for a medical condition quickly because he mistrusts the system in which the care is offered. He may not have access to healthcare due to the disparities in income or available resources in his region. He may choose to avoid contact with any healthcare professional because he is afraid that due to his immigration status he may be refused treatment or deported.

In residences with people from varied backgrounds there are real challenges for a person of color. The threat of discrimination and bigotry exists in the world, so of course, this holds true within residences. What happens if a black woman and a racist white woman are made to share a room? Are staff looking out for this when they pair up residents? Is the black woman physically and emotionally safe or living in fear?

If a Hispanic man "isolates" himself in his room, will he be deemed "non-social" and left alone? What if his isolation is based on his disconnection with the normative activities that don't match with his own cultural experiences? What if English is his second language and as his dementia progresses, he can no longer understand and engage with the English speakers who surround him?

If a black or brown woman is used to her needs being ignored by the healthcare system, will she feel comfortable pressing the call button to ask for help? Can she be assured that the staff who are there to comfort her will take care of her? I hate to say it, but I have witnessed racism amongst colleagues despite professional and ethical guidelines to which we all should adhere.

We must remember that many people of color have experienced long and repeated racism and inequality throughout their entire lives. This has left a mark on their soul, a trauma, that can play a part in how they view and respond to aging. We must understand that this could lead to mistrust toward healthcare professionals and others who are trying to support them. We must do our best, as families and professionals, to ask the hard questions, listen without judgment to the answers, and be prepared to respond, adapt, and provide equitable, compassionate support.

Mental Illness

This is something very close to my heart. I was diagnosed with a generalized anxiety disorder in my late 20s. I have spent the last 20 years learning how to manage my symptoms, which first emerged when I was just three years old. My anxiety, although more manageable than in the past, still presents itself periodically and with a force and power that can knock me down. I fully expect that as I age my anxiety will impact the way in which I face potential illness or other challenges of aging.

According to the World Health Organization, one in four people are affected by a mental illness or neurological disorder. Despite the prevalence of mental illness and the impact it can have on a person's functioning, the stigma and shame associated with having a mental illness runs deep. Not only do people avoid seeking treatment, others (even healthcare professionals) judge a person as being responsible for their emotional functioning. In spite of scientific evidence that brain chemistry can lead to mental illness—as can unavoidable environmental factors, life stressors, illness, and trauma—those suffering with a mental illness are too often blamed and shamed.

What does this mean for the older adult population? A few things. As I mentioned earlier, if a man or woman loses a spouse or moves into a retirement residence (or any other change) and depression or anxiety follows, many will nonchalantly brush it off as "normal" and not intervene to help. Without support, depression or anxiety can deepen and interfere with a person's ability to care for himself or herself. It must be addressed.

Many mental illnesses are chronic, beginning for some, like me, in early childhood, or for others in their teens or early 20s. Many of these people learn over the years to manage their symptoms and function well. Others struggle for a lifetime. Regardless of one's lifetime experience with a mental illness, when a person gets older there are natural fears and questions that emerge such as

"How will I die?" "Will I be in pain?" "Will I be alone?" "Will my family support me?" For someone with a pre-existing mental illness, these questions can take on another level of power within a person's emotional and psychological well-being (which can lead to physical problems).

I do not doubt that I will have periods of increased anxiety as I age. Fear and doubt creep into my mind daily about all sorts of things, and it has taken years for me to develop tools to combat these internal battles. As I age I imagine that I will become more afraid of life and what is in front of me. I will need my family (my kids when they are adults) to ensure that my anxiety is managed and that I am provided with the appropriate support to ensure that I don't live in a state of panic so that whatever good parts of my life are still present are not lost to me.

Mental illness is powerful. It deserves proper care and attention equal to the support we provide to people with a physical illness.

Share the Story

Many healthcare professionals will not think to ask questions related to someone's experience with trauma, abuse, or discrimination. It is up to us to advocate for these groups and to educate those around them who are providing support. All individuals, including those with special considerations, deserve to have family and healthcare providers demonstrate empathy and skill in making sure that their history is considered in the development of their treatment plans, living arrangements, and the delivery of care.

Conclusion

Spark. Ignite. Launch.

If you picked up this book, the aging process is something you think about. Perhaps you're a family caregiver and you want to absorb all of the information available to help you in your role as a caregiver. Maybe you're in your mid-70s and you're trying to ensure that you and your family are prepared for whatever lies ahead. Or maybe you're a healthcare professional on a quest to understand how you can adjust and improve your approach with patients and advance the system in which you work.

However this book fell into your lap, my hope is that something in these pages sparked and ignited a fire that launches you into a personal mission to do things differently. To have proactive conversations. To see yourself and others as a whole person. To demand more from the healthcare professionals and system. To insist on a collaborative care approach. To build a team with common goals.

I know it's not easy to change your ways. It can be scary and uncomfortable. But I know, deep down, that any discomfort now will produce long-term results that will bring peace and comfort to you and your family for years to come.

The time is now.

Resources

Thank you for reading this book. I hope that it brought you value and provided insight, ideas, and inspiration to change the way you understand and plan for aging. If you are looking for additional tools or guidance from me, please visit my website, www.stephanierickson.ca. You can find toolkits, a blog, and videos, as well as a tele-consulting program that addresses aging, caregiving, and overall health and well-being. You can also connect with me on social media:

Instagram – @stephericksonhost

Facebook – Stephanie Erickson, Media Commentator, Family Caregiving Expert

Twitter – @FamCareExpert

LinkedIn – Stephanie Erickson

Additional resources:

Free healthcare proxy forms state by state (U.S.):
https://www.aarp.org/caregiving/financial-legal/free-printable-advance-directives/

Free healthcare planning forms province by province (Canada): https://www.dyingwithdignity.ca/download_your_advance_care_planning_kit

National Alliance for Caregiving
https://www.caregiving.org

Family Caregiver Alliance
https://www.caregiver.org

Carers Canada
https://www.carerscanada.ca

Alzheimer's Society of Canada
https://alzheimer.ca/en/Home

Alzheimer's Association (U.S.)
https://www.alz.org

Glossary of Terms

Below are some general definitions of different types of senior living environments. Keep in mind, however, that there are nuances from state to state and province to province. In some regions a level of care may refer to one thing, yet in the state just next door that same term describes a different level of care. It is for this reason I use the general term "residence" throughout this book.

Retirement Communities/Senior Communities – This term refers to environments for active and autonomous seniors. They are not included as part of the description of "residences" used throughout this book.

Assisted Living Facility/Assisted Living/Assisted Living Community – An environment for seniors who require services to maintain a certain level of autonomy. Services are usually related to medication administration, hygiene care, meal preparation, and domestic assistance. Some level of nursing care is available around the clock for individuals who do not require medical care. Often in these environments the rooms are structured as apartments, some with their own bathroom and half kitchens, which may include a microwave, sink, and refrigerator. A person who lives here may be able to prepare a simple meal, such as toast or coffee. In this environment, the person does not require 24/7 supervision.

Board and Care/Residential Care Home – An environment that is within a residential neighborhood. These homes are smaller and generally house two to fifteen individuals. Private and shared rooms are available and most have shared bathrooms. The care provided is the same as within an assisted living facility (see above), but because the setting is smaller (less space) the person would not have a small refrigerator or toaster.

Long-term Care Facility – An environment in which individuals require continuous care and supervision. The rooms do not have a half kitchen and can be shared or private. The bathroom may be private or shared as well. In this environment, individuals are not able to meet their needs independently. Often within these facilities, there is a separate secured area (locked) for individuals with dementia, or if the symptoms are manageable, the person may remain in the general population. In these facilities, there will be a doctor who is available periodically on-site but by phone around the clock. There will always be a licensed nurse (RN, LPN, RNA) and they may have other professionals available as well, such as a social worker or physiotherapist. In some of these environments, skilled-nursing care, such as catheter care or injections are offered.

Skilled Nursing Facility – An environment for patients who require medical and nursing care by licensed professionals. This can be for short-term or long-term stays. It is very similar to a hospital-type environment in which many professionals offer services (occupational therapy, social work, nursing, etc.). These higher services include things like catheter care, injections, IV therapy, etc. Not all long-term care environments offer skilled nursing care services.

Nursing Home – A term used in the past that refers to what is now called a long-term care facility (see above).

Memory Care – For individuals who have dementia, they will at some point require 24/7 supervision, which can be offered in a secured setting. At times, this setting is an extension of an assisted or long-term care facility. In a memory care setting, there will always be a licensed nurse (RN, LPN, RNA) and they may have other professionals available as well, such as a social worker or physiotherapist. The setting will have visits from an MD weekly (at least) and will have access to a MD on-call.

Rehabiliation Facility – A person stays in a rehab facility when they have short-term medical and skilled-nursing care needs. For example, after a hip surgery a person may be sent to rehabilitation for a three-week period to gain strength and access auxiliary services, such as occupational therapy and physiotherapy. In these facilities, there will be individuals of all ages.

Acknowledgments

Throughout my career as a social worker I have met amazing people. I have been honoured, time and again, to be included in their lives in their most vulnerable moments. It is for all of you that I write this book and express my deepest respect and gratitude. To the many colleagues I have who are knee deep in this fight for change alongside me, thank you. We can do this.

I couldn't have completed this project without the support of many dedicated and talented professionals. Thank you to my publishing team, Debra Englander (editor), Christy Collins (Constellation Book Services – design and layout), David Aretha (proofreader), Hendrik Dimter (online marketing) and Jessie Huard (administrative assistant). I am grateful for your keen eyes and creativity. To my publishing consultant, Martha Bullen (Bullen Publishing Services), my gratitude extends beyond your skills and knowledge of the publishing process. When I felt discouraged, you reminded me of the value of this book and the power and authenticity of my voice. You gave me the confidence I needed to put this out into the world. Thank you, Martha. I am so grateful for your expertise, advice, and support.

It's not only my publishing team that deserves thanks and recognition.

To the readers who offered their time to give this manuscript a first read and share their thoughts all I can say is, "Wow." I'm humbled that you took your own personal time to support me and this movement for change. Thank you: Stuart Furman, Sandra Robbins, Nancy Christianson Beyak, Susan Sofer, Sabrina Dion, Dr. Elise Levinoff, Dr. Serge Gauthier, Charles Sabatino, Trisha Felgar, Dr. Sharon Cohen, Miverva Maharajh, April Hayward, Areta Lloyd, Todd Looney, Mandy Novak-Leonard, Lauren Snedeker, Georgia Papadopoulos, Michelle Olson and Jana Bartley.

To my dear friend Sandra, you have been my sounding board more times than I can count. Your balanced and reasonable perspective on all things professional and personal helped to steady my nerves and gave me confidence to forge ahead. I love you, Glitter Mama.

To my flying friends, you have no idea how our trainings contributed to the completion of this book. The laughs, (my) tears, and the physical effort put into those trainings are my stress antidote and free me up to fly back into the work. Thank you, especially à ma gang de vieux, Patrick, Annie and Isabelle. You bring me courage, comfort and laughs. Fly high. Fly safe. Fly free. I love you all.

To Jagger, my furriest friend, thank you for keeping my toes warm as I sat for hours at the computer. Your tail wags and frequent requests for hugs kept me sane and calm.

To my family, the original source of life lessons and inspirations, thank you for building the foundation of what has become my personal and professional success. You have shown me, first hand, about the values and actions that lead to living well and aging well.

Grandma Mickey, thank you for teaching me the importance of family, community and connection. Grandma Betty, thank you for showing me how quietness and observation are valuable and wonderful ways to appreciate and soak in what is around you. Papa, thank you for showing me how essential it is to live passionately and create and embrace life's adventures while you can.

Mom, thank you for helping me learn about forgiveness and the power it holds in moving beyond what paralyzes us. Dad, I miss you every day and wish you could be here to celebrate this accomplishment with me. You taught me about taking responsibility, expressing remorse without shame and at any cost, and how patience and time can rebuild a relationship into a solid and meaningful one. And to Lisa, my sister, my confidant and show-stopping best friend, you are everything. We managed the worst crisis of our lives as partners with unyielding trust. This shows me how much can be done well, even in the worst of times. What we have together is unique, a true always-by-your-side, non-judgmental, you're-never-alone bond that feeds my soul and makes me laugh like no other.

To my kids, Charlotte and Maxime, thank you for understanding the importance of my work and appreciating the time and emotional energy I needed to devote to this. It is my love for you both, and your futures, that fills me up daily and inspires me to make this world a better place. You are my hearts. You are the source of my energy, drive, and love in all that I do. I love you both so much it hurts (and causes me to cry with joy daily.)

And lastly, to my husband, Philippe, thank you for listening, ad nauseum, to the challenges and excitement of this process.

You have cheered me on and have always supported my entrepreneurial spirit to get out of my comfort zone, push myself and try new things in order to make a difference in people's lives in any way I can (even if it's picking up trash in the street during our walks). My partner in life and love. My best friend. I love you.

About the Author

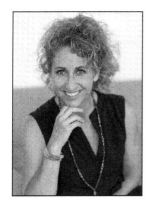

STEPHANIE ERICKSON, author of *Plan for Aging Well*, was born and raised in California. She has a Master's Degree in Social Work, is a Certified Alzheimer's Disease Treatment Specialist (CADTS) and is licensed in both Quebec and California.

She founded Erickson Resource Group, a clinical practice providing decision-making capacity evaluations for legal proceedings and expert opinions related to support for older adults. She also provides online consulting services for caregivers throughout North America. As a Family Caregiving Expert, she is a regular contributor on media outlets throughout the U.S. and Canada discussing topics related to caregiving, health and well-being.

Stephanie is passionate about sharing her experience and knowledge and encouraging others to take control of their health and advocate on behalf of vulnerable populations. As a mom and entrepreneur, free time is hard to find. Yet, Stephanie always carves out time to train on the flying trapeze. She lives in Montreal with her husband, two children and energetic golden retriever.

You can learn more about Stephanie at:
www.stephanieerickson.ca or find her on
Instagram – @stephericksonhost
Facebook – Stephanie Erickson, Media Commentator,
Family Caregiving Expert
Twitter – @FamCareExpert
LinkedIn – Stephanie Erickson

Made in the USA
Columbia, SC
27 September 2020

21582801R00104